Fascinomas -Fascinating Medical Myst
Clifton K. Meador, M.D.

"Fascinomas" are fascinating by their very nature; they are stories that illustrate the reasoning of the master diagnostician faced with the complexities of daunting clinical challenges... They are object lessons in the essence of the shared journey between patient and physician: both are immersed in a particular clinical narrative, both hope for insights that can solve the illness experience, both try to fathom the idioms each contributes to the dialogue, and both are committed to this trusting alliance... Every patient is his or her own fascinoma.

Nortin M. Hadler MD MACP MACR FACOEM
Professor of Medicine and Microbiology/Immunology
University of North Carolina School of Medicine
Author of The Last Well Person, Worried Sick, Stabbed in the Back, Rethinking Aging, and Citizen Patient

Clifton Meador is a superb story-teller who has been teaching and practicing medicine for more than 50 years. He knows how to "plot" a Medical Mystery. At the same time, he reveals how some of our best doctors arrive at the right diagnosis the old-fashioned way-by listening to their patients.

His experience has taught him that touching, asking questions, listening, and truly "seeing" the patient are the sensory arts that may be lost if physicians become too dependent on "reading" tests. His tales tell us what health care reformers mean when they talk about "patient-centered medicine."

Maggie Mahar
Author of Money Driven Medicine
Editor of Healthbeatblog.

Using a simple and direct language, Dr. Meador delivers charm, wit, and always surprising stories that carry fundamental teachings dedicated to the best service to the patients and the profession. I have been reading his books with great delight since the 1990's, and have enjoyed translating them into Spanish for discussions with my students. The curious cases he presents in his books underscore how difficult it can be to reach the proper diagnosis and the right treatment without the dedication of true doctors.

Ximena Páez M.D.
Professor
Laboratory of Behavioral Physiology
School of Medicine
Universidad de los Andes
Mérida-Venezuela

Fascinating
Fascinomas
Medical Mysteries

ISBN: 1491029277

ISBN 13: 9781491029275

Library of Congress Control Number: 2013913504

CreateSpace Independent Publishing Platform

North Charleston, South Carolina

Other Books
by Clifton K. Meador, M.D.

A Little Book of Doctors' Rules, Hanley & Belfus, 1992

With R. H. Lanius, A Little Book of Nurses' Rules, Hanley & Belfus, 1993

With W. Wadlington, Pearls from a Pediatric Practice, Hanley & Belfus, 1998

A Little Book of Doctors' Rules II, A Compilation, Hanley & Belfus, 1999

With C. M. Slovis and K. D. Wrenn, A Little Book of Emergency Medicine Rules, Hanley & Belfus, 2000

With W. Wadlington and M. Howington, How to Raise Healthy and Happy Children, iUniverse, 2001

Med School, Hillsboro Press, Providence Publishing Corporation, 2003

Symptoms of Unknown Origin, A Medical Odyssey, Vanderbilt University Press, 2005

Twentieth Century Men in Medicine: Personal Reflections, iUniverse, 2007

Puzzling Symptoms: How to Solve the Puzzle of Your Symptoms, Cable Publishing, 2008

Med School, Revised Edition, Cable Publishing, 2009

True Medical Detective Stories, CreateSpace, 2012

Fascinating

Fascinomas

Medical Mysteries

Clifton K. Meador, M.D.
Author of True Medical Detective Stories

Table of Contents

Fascinomas – fascinating medical mysteries

Foreword

Fascinoma combines the words "fascinate" with "oma." The suffix "oma" usually denotes a growth or tumor. The Merriam-Webster Collegiate Dictionary defines fascinating as "to be irresistibly attractive or to command the interest of or to be extremely interesting." Thus a fascinoma is medical slang for an unusually interesting medical case.

Fascinomas are patient stories that are indelibly stored in the minds of physicians. They are stories told over and over in hospital medical lounges. Every physician has at least one fascinoma to tell.

Following publication of True Medical Detective Stories this past year, I have been flooded with requests for more patient stories. True Medical Detective Stories was dedicated to the memory of Berton Roueche', noted writer for the New Yorker and the creator of the genre of medical detective stories. There were 19 patient stories in the book, most of which were solved by listening and talking.

Fascinomas, in most cases, are also medical detective stories. They often require some special effort by the patient or the physician or both to unravel the underlying causes. The causes of the illness may be obscure or rare or even unheard of before. Many fascinomas are so rare they are one time occurrences – unique to the particular patient. Some, as you will read, are self inflicted.

Over the past year I have asked colleagues to share patient stories with me. This book is a compilation of 35 such medical mysteries or fascinomas. Nearly all emphasize the need for the physician to hear and understand the life narrative of the patient. They reinforce the old dictum that it is as important to know the patient with the disease as it is to know the disease.

My method in writing these patient stories has been to stick very closely to the clinical story and facts. By facts I mean all symptoms, physical findings, laboratory findings, and results of any imaging studies; these are all true. All of the patient identifiers have been changed. None of the patient names are true nor are any of the geographic details accurate. All have been altered to protect the privacy of the patient.

Some of the physicians allowed me to use their real names in the stories. All of the other physicians' names are fictitious. At the end of each chapter, the physician who shared the clinical facts is identified.

Acknowledgements.

Many friends, colleagues, and physicians have contributed to this book.

I want to thank especially those physicians who have shared patient stories or who made editorial suggestions and comments about the manuscript. These physicians are Paul Barnett, Sidney R. Block, Jack Fisher, Robert Foote, Rand Fredericksen, Alan Graber, Jim Jirjis, Lloyd King, Robert Latham, John Newman, Ximena Paez, Alan Siegal, Betty Ruth Speir, William Stoney, Curt Tribble, Will Van Derveer, Larry Wolff, and Michael Zanoli.

I appreciate the suggestions or editorial comments of Virginia Fuqua-Meadows and my daughter Mary Kathleen Meador. I am thankful for the encouragement from Dr. Nortin Hadler and Maggie Mahar. My classmate Dr. Oscar Crofford and his wife Jane made many helpful suggestions.

I especially appreciate the superb editing job done by Beth Stein. She added so much to the telling of the stories.

And most of all I appreciate the support and editorial comments of my wife Ann Cowden Meador.

Cover Design:
Mark Cowden
Nashville

Chapter One

A Puzzling Paralysis *

Being clumsy is one of the many unfortunate symptoms that often plagues young teenagers. But when Julia Wilkinson began bumping into furniture with some regularity, her mother Marie took note.

It was just a week after Julia turned 13. The healthy adolescent had celebrated the milestone with family and friends on a warm July evening. But in the past few days, Marie had begun to notice what she thought was more than a typical lack of coordination on Julia's part. When her normally careful daughter dropped a bowl at dinner, shattering it on the floor, Marie became concerned.

She asked Julia to walk in a straight line across the room from one wall to the other. The request seemed silly to the 13-year old, but Julia complied. She began tracing an imaginary line towards the kitchen counter.

It only took a few steps to see something was seriously wrong: Julia was swaying dramatically from left to right. Unable to maintain her balance, she fell to the floor. The family left dinner on the table and rushed Julia to the emergency room of the University Hospital.

When the Wilkinsons came through the big glass doors of the ER supporting and practically dragging Julia, the first person they encountered was Dr. James Reese, the senior resident in the ER. Dr. Reese went into full action, guiding the threesome into the closest exam room.

Julia was now barely able to move her feet. Dr. Reese quickly assessed her neurological status, noting absent tendon reflexes in both legs and definite weakness in her foot and thigh muscles. Julia's arms and upper body strength remained normal, however, and there was no loss of feeling to touch or pin prick. The findings suggested an ascending paralysis, most often associated with Guillain-Barre syndrome. Polio would also have been a consideration in years past.

Guillain-Barre syndrome is an uncommon disorder that causes the immune system to attack the peripheral nervous system (PNS). The PNS nerves connect the brain and spinal cord with the rest of the body. Damage to these nerves makes it difficult for them to transmit signals, so the muscles have trouble responding to the brain. No one knows what causes the syndrome. Sometimes it is triggered by an infection, surgery or a vaccination.

Immediately, Dr. Reese ordered a series of tests. A CT scan of Julia's brain and spinal cord was normal, as were the blood chemistries and examination of her urine. A spinal tap revealed completely normal spinal fluid, ruling out a number of infectious causes including all forms of meningitis. It also ruled out Guillain-Barre.

Dr. Max Wellborn was senior attending physician in the ER. He and Dr. Reese began reviewing his long list of possible causes for Julia's ascending paralysis. One by one, they ordered the remaining tests and procedures to rule out each cause on the list.

With no immediate explanation for Julia's ascending paralysis, she was admitted to the Intensive Care Unit (ICU) for close monitoring. A ventilator was brought bedside for possible artificial ventilation, since breathing would become difficult or absent should the paralysis involve her chest muscles. In a few hours, Julia noted weakness in her arms and shoulders but could still move them. Meanwhile, her bewildered parents spent a sleepless night in the ICU waiting room.

The next morning when pediatric residents made their 7 a.m. rounds, they were astounded to see Julia sitting on the edge of the bed swinging her feet back and forth. Grinning broadly, she got up and wobbled towards them. She held the edge of the bed to steady herself, but the near full recovery was miraculous.

The evening nurse told residents that at every neuro check during the night there was more and more unexplained return of strength to Julia's legs and arms. When Dr. Wellborn caught up with the residents' group, he was smiling.

"I know the etiology of Julia's paralysis and also what cured her," Wellborn said. "My conversation just now with Ms. Toll, the evening nurse, was the key. She told me the intervention she made last night. Anyone care to guess?"

The residents looked completely puzzled. No one ventured a guess.

Wellborn continued. "Last night, Ms. Toll noticed a small lump deep in Julia's hair behind her right ear. On closer inspection, it was a swollen tick, which the nurse promptly removed. Although Ms. Toll had no idea she had initiated the cure of the paralysis, that's precisely what happened: Julia is recovering from Tick Paralysis. Julia had no idea about the hidden bite, so it was pure luck — and a nurse's careful attention to detail — that the tick was found and removed."

Neither Max Wellborn nor any of the residents had ever heard of Tick Paralysis. "I didn't even have Tick Paralysis on my list. I had to look it up," the doctor confessed. "But I'll never miss that again."

Tick Paralysis is a different disease from the more common tick-borne diseases Rocky Mountain Spotted Fever, Erlichiosis or Lyme Disease. These are infectious diseases with the infectious agent injected via the saliva of the tick. The infecting agents are classified as a Rickettsia. The same species of ticks that transmit these infections can also transmit a nerve toxin that caused Julia's paralysis, but in a different fashion

With Tick Paralysis, if the tick remains attached to the human for several days, the salivary gland of the tick produces a nerve toxin. This nerve toxin is then secreted into the human and produces an ascending paralysis. The nerve toxin has a very short half life so that removal of the tick leads to a rapid recovery in an average of one and a half days. The disease is worldwide and probably transmitted by over 40 species of ticks. (1) Some wild animals also become paralyzed and die from the toxin.

The incidence of Tick Paralysis in humans is unknown. Most would classify it as a rare cause of ascending paralysis. The reason tick paralysis is rare is that the ticks usually fall off or are removed before secreting the nerve toxin. One meta-analysis of the medical literature found only 50 reported cases in a 60-year period. If the tick is not removed, the mortality rate can be as high as 6 to 10 percent, death coming from respiratory failure. Since the advent of ventilators, the death rate is probably below 6 percent.

Young girls seem to be more susceptible to Tick Paralysis, because they favor long hair — the perfect cover for marauding ticks. In Julia's case, the nurse's discovery produced the cure unwittingly, which proves that serendipity can be the only source of evidence in some medical mysteries.

+ When faced with a patient with an ascending paralysis, the physician detective must consider a large number of possibilities; acute peripheral nerve inflammation after infection with Campylobacter; porphyria, a defect in hemoglobin synthesis; periodic paralysis from low or high blood potassium; organophosphate insecticide poisoning; heavy metal poisoning from arsenic or mercury; Elapid snake bites; botulism from food poisoning; psychogenic hysterical paralysis; Marine fish poisonings; and of course Tick Paralysis.

**This case was shared by:*

Dr. Jim Jirjis, MD MBA
Assistant Chief Medical Officer for Vanderbilt Medical Group
Assistant Professor of Medicine
Department of Medicine, Vanderbilt University School of Medicine.

Chapter Two

A Sticky Situation *

Ethyl Snodgrass and her husband Grady came together for their visits to see Dr. Paul Barnett. Ethyl called Grady "Big Daddy," and Grady called Ethyl "Little Mama."

Big Daddy and Little Mama lived on a small farm about 30 miles from town. Both were in their early 60s and in general good health, except for their shared weight problems. Big Daddy called it their "acute and chronic biscuit intoxication."

Ethyl was genuinely interested in losing weight and asked the doctor about a diet. Grady, on the other hand, could not have cared less. He was certainly no help. "In fact, the older I get, the more meat I like on my women," he said with a hearty laugh. Ethyl swatted him playfully and rolled her eyes.

After a normal baseline workup, both patients met with a dietician and an exercise trainer to set up a healthy weight loss program they could follow. Dr. Barnett talked to them about expectations and some challenges of dieting and warned them about products that promised fast weight loss. He stressed especially the danger of diet pills and told the Snodgrass's to stay away from those.

About a week after starting the reduced calorie diet, Ethyl called Barnett. She had started to have diarrhea daily, reporting frequent, large volume, almost liquid bowel movements. Barnett thought perhaps too much roughage in their healthier diet was the culprit, so he told her to cut back. The diarrhea continued. Barnett then launched a full diarrhea workup including multiple stool cultures, checks for ova and parasites, a colonoscopy, small bowel x-rays and multiple blood tests for malabsorption studies. All test results were normal. The diarrhea continued, now even worse in frequency and volume.

Frustrated, Barnett had the couple come in for a review of the history. They sat down in his office and began going over in detail the last few weeks. Ethyl said the diet had been a big change for both of them and she found herself hungry much of the time. With that, she took a stick of gum from her purse and began to chew. She told Barnett it helped the cravings.

Grady said he had no diarrhea, which ruled out any infection at work. Other than grumbling about how much he missed his favorite foods, he had no physical complaints. As Grady talked, Ethyl kept putting one stick of gum after another in her mouth. She realized Barnett was watching her unwrap yet another piece and suddenly remembered her manners. "Want a stick?" she asked, holding out the package. That's when he saw the world "sugarless" on the label. A light bulb came on in his mind.

"That stuff has sorbital. How much do you chew a day?" he asked.

"Oh, 'bout 10 packs." Ethyl answered. Grady nodded agreement.

"It's no wonder you have diarrhea," Barnett said. "Sorbital is not absorbed in the intestines and it pulls huge amounts of water into the gut. It's almost like an internal enema."

Sugarless gum is a well known cause of diarrhea when chewed in large amounts of more than 6 or 7 sticks a day. Each stick has around one and a half grams of sorbital. The non-absorbability of the sorbital causes a shift of water into the gut. The large volume of water is quickly passed down the intestine causing the watery diarrhea.

"But I like the sweet taste," Ethyl protested. "I kept hoping it would help me not eat so much, so I could lose weight."

Barnett said he sympathized, but no more sugarless gum for her — period.

Grady could only say, "Well I'll be. Well I'll be." As the two toddled out of the office, he kept elbowing Ethyl, "Little Mama, I told you that you was chewing too much gum. I told you."

Case shared by:

Paul Barnett, M.D.
Associate Clinical Professor of Medicine
Department of Medicine
Vanderbilt University School of Medicine".

Chapter Three

*The Cause of Some Symptoms Can Be Illusory**

Veronica Settler had been coughing up blood for more than a year when she went in to see Dr. William Stoney. Stoney was a noted thoracic and cardiac surgeon, known both for his surgical skill and his ability to sort through difficult cases.

Mrs. Settler had been referred to Stoney by a family physician in Arkansas. Despite all of his diagnostic efforts, he couldn't find the cause for the bloody sputum.

Mrs. Settler described her coughing up blood as intermittent and unpredictable. Sometimes she would go for over a month and then cough up blood daily for a week or more. She had no fever and her general health was excellent.

She had married her high school sweetheart, an outstanding halfback on the local team with all-state honors. Randy Settler went on to the University of Arkansas, where he and Veronica got married. The year was 1978, about the same time she began coughing up blood. Mrs. Settler was 23 years old at the time.

Dr. Stoney admitted Mrs. Settler and began to repeat all the tests that might identify the cause for bleeding somewhere in her lungs and bronchial tubes. He even considered vicarious menstruation and sought a gynecological consultation. Vicarious menstruation occurs when uterine tissue somehow gets implanted in the nose or bronchus. At the time of monthly menstruation, the aberrant tissues also bleed, giving a puzzling periodic bleeding. Mrs. Settler, herself, had wondered if the bloody sputum might be close to her monthly menstrual periods. But the sputum was examined microscopically and no uterine or other aberrant tissue was found – another blind diagnostic alley.

Mrs. Settler's chest x-ray showed a large calcified lymph node sitting next to the trachea and right bronchial tube. These were the days before CT scans or MRIs, so a bronchoscope was the best tool. But repeated looks down the bronchoscope by several doctors revealed nothing that looked like a tumor or a bleeding site on the inside of the trachea or right bronchus.

Stoney had several colleagues review the chest x-rays with him. The consensus of the consultants was that it would make sense to remove the calcified node, since it could represent an active fungus infection such as histoplasmosis, a prevalent fungus in Arkansas and the Ohio and Mississippi Valleys. Some thought it could even be a low-grade malignant tumor or a tumor of the lymph nodes. Whatever it was, its close proximity to the airways could conceivably lead to periodic erosions and bleeding.

Dr. Stoney met with Mrs. Settler and her husband and offered to do an exploratory thoracotomy (open chest operation) to remove the large node or mass. The couple wanted time to think it over and asked to be discharged from the hospital.

A month later, Mrs. Settler was admitted and had the thoracotomy done by Dr. Stoney. The node was easily removed. Tissue examination showed what appeared to be an old and healed fungus infection with histoplasmosis. There was no evidence at surgery for active invasion of the air tubes by the lymph node. The operation did not uncover the cause for the bloody sputum. Mrs. Settler went home on the 8th post-op day.

Three weeks after the operation, Mrs. Settler called Dr. Stoney to tell him she had been coughing up blood for over a week, this time in large quantities. She was worried about the amount of blood she was losing in her sputum. Stoney insisted she come immediately to the hospital for admission. He was at a complete loss as to what he would do. In his wildest thoughts, he would do a complete clotting workup. Maybe he had missed some weird hemophilia bleeding disorder? But that didn't make much sense since there was no bleeding problem from the thoracotomy.

Mrs. Settler was admitted to the hospital, still spitting up almost pure blood in her sputum. In the 1970s, there were still four-bed units in many hospitals, called "semiprivate beds." Mrs. Settler was admitted to such a unit. Each bed had its own curtain to pull around and provide some privacy.

When Dr. Stoney made his morning rounds the next day, he saw out of the corner of his eye the woman in the adjacent bed making signs by nodding her head, indicating she wanted to speak with Stoney privately. The woman got out of her bed and walked into the hallway, waiting for him to finish with Mrs. Settler. When he exited, she grabbed his arm and whispered into his ear, "She's sticking her gums with needles to make them bleed." She turned abruptly and went back to her bed.

Stoney examined Mrs. Settler's mouth and found multiple small cuts in the far reaches of her gums behind the back molars, some still bleeding. It became clear she had self-inflicted the wounds and made up the entire story, submitting herself to an unnecessary and life-threatening operation. She was continuing to make needle cuts to get medical and other attention.

Stoney was not sure of his next move. He called for her husband to join him and Mrs. Settler in the small consultation room off of the lobby. He had a nurse attend the meeting as a witness.

Dr. Stony then told in detail all that he had done to find the cause for the bloody sputum and his reasons for doing the chest surgery. Then he told them what Mrs. Settler had done to fool and mislead the efforts by self-inflicting the bleeding. He let them know in detail that he knew about the needles and the dangers of what Mrs. Settler had done. He waited a few moments for Mr. or Mrs. Settler to respond. Neither said a word. Both sat there with blank expressions. Stoney pressed for comments. Both only shook their heads. Neither responded.

In order to bring some closure to his own frustrations, Stoney had a novel solution. He had brought a pint of a cough syrup with him. He told Mrs. Settler to take a teaspoon of the cough syrup each morning until she finished the entire bottle. "If you do this, then the bloody sputum will go away," he told her in his most serious voice. He estimated the syrup would last about six months. Stoney, lacking any real cure, thought the use of the cough syrup would give Mrs. Settler an out, an excuse or reason to stop her self- infliction. Stoney then left the room and never saw Mrs. Settler again.

The story of Mrs. Settler went all over the doctors' lounge for weeks. Every one wondered if Stoney's almost hypnotic suggestion would work.

Almost six months to the day, Stoney got a call from a doctor in Melbourne, Arkansas. He said that he was now Mrs. Settler's family doctor. She had told him about the chest operation and her history of coughing up blood. He wanted any clinical details Stoney had to share. Stoney told him the entire story.

As an afterthought, Stoney asked, "What is she seeing you about?"

The local doctor hesitated a moment, then said, "Your information has been helpful, but I'm not sure what I will do with it. She's been urinating bloody urine for several weeks but with no demonstrable lesion in her bladder or kidneys."

Stoney only shook his head, wondering what drove Mrs. Settler and all like her to do what they do to themselves.

The most puzzling problems faced by physicians are those that are self-inflicted or feigned. According to Marc Feldman, M.D., a recognized international expert, there are four types of self-harm: Munchausen Syndrome, Munchausen by Proxy, Malingering, and Factitious Disorder.

Munchausen Syndrome was named after Baron von Munchausen, an 18th century German aristocrat known for his tall, elaborate tales. Munchausen himself was not sick. Patients with Munchausen Syndrome inflict real harm by injecting feces, bleeding themselves, injecting insulin, taking anticoagulants or feigning serious neurological symptoms. The list of self-inflictions is long. These patients are quite dramatic and move from one emergency room to another and from town to town fooling one doctor after another. They do what they do to get attention not available from normal social encounters. The condition is considered to be a psychiatric disorder.

Mrs. Settler was very private in her self-induced bleeding; she would not be considered to have Munchausen Syndrome.

Munchausen by Proxy is when one person inflicts harm on another person. Most often it's a mother inflicting harm on one of her children. This is a crime and should be reported to police.

Malingering is conscious infliction or feigning of an illness for drugs or monetary or other tangible gain. Malingering often co-exists with a borderline or antisocial personality. Mrs. Settler was not seeking any tangible gain.

The fourth type of self-harm is called a Factitious Disorder. Patients with this disorder do not move from place to place and they are not dramatic in their presentation. Many lead quiet and, to some extent, productive lives. They are seeking some sort of attention otherwise not available in their daily lives. Mrs. Settler was a typical example of a Factitious Disorder. Most of these people are incurable.

All of these disorders are difficult and usually impossible to manage. One essential feature of the doctor-patient relationship is the requirement for trust. When trust is consciously violated, there can be no successful encounter with a physician. These patients, once discovered, will move immediately to another physician. Such was the case with Mrs. Settler.

Case shared by:

William Stoney, M.D.
Professor of Cardiac and Thoracic Surgery, Emeritus
Vanderbilt University School of Medicine

Chapter Four

Seasonal Disorder *

Fred Altman was a happy-go-lucky traveling salesman with a lovely wife, two young boys he adored and overall good health — except twice this month he had been admitted to the University Hospital with severe headaches.

"This was the worst headache I ever had in my whole life," Altman said. "Not like the kind of headache you get from driving all day with the sun in your eyes. I've had those, too. But this was something different — much, much worse."

With the headaches came nausea and vomiting. On both occasions when the pain started, Fred became dizzy and confused. It was November and he was looking forward to traveling during the holidays, but he worried that one of these awful headaches might hit him again with his family in the car.

A careful medical history revealed Altman had also experienced these same symptoms in late March of the same year, but these were much milder and lasted only an hour. He didn't seek medical attention, chalking it up to perhaps a few too many cocktails the previous weekends. He had experienced no recurrences of the headache or other symptoms until the two hospital admissions, the first on November 21st and the second on November 30th.

On both admissions, Altman underwent extensive diagnostic workups. The careful and thorough physical examinations proved normal. Neither his blood pressure nor other vital signs fluctuated throughout his stays. Head and spine CT scans were also normal on the first admission, and an MRI of his brain was normal on the second admission. All routine blood chemistry tests were normal. Furthermore, within 24 hours of being admitted to the hospital both times, Altman was symptom free.

Other than his history of symptoms, there was no objective abnormal finding by any means. Several members of the residency team were beginning to wonder about psychological or stress causes for the headaches. But Altman and his wife insisted life was good in every way. He loved his job and family and couldn't point to anything extraordinary or stressful.

Walker Evans, the chief medical resident, called in Simpkins Jackson, a consultant in Neurology. Dr. Jackson was well known for taking very careful medical histories and solving complex cases.

After spending more than an hour with Altman Dr. Jackson said, "Here is all I know about Fred's recurring illness: He had one severe episode in March and a couple of minor ones in early April, then no more until these two admissions in November. All summer long he enjoyed vigorous good health, swimming and golfing, shooting to a handicap of seven, as a matter of fact.

"Whatever this is, it does not occur in the summer. It is some kind of early spring and fall recurring illness. I asked him every known pollen-grass-seed-dust-pollution question I could think of. He is a traveling salesmen delivering and taking orders from small grocery stores and gas stations, selling candies, crackers, and small edible items. Stops every few miles across the country roads out from towns. I even asked him if he ate different candies before the episodes, trying to get something to correlate with the seasonal headaches. Nothing so far. By the way, all the headaches came on late in the afternoon."

Just one week after Altman was discharged from the last November hospital stay, he was back. This time, he arrived by ambulance. He was unconscious and unresponsive to painful stimulation, with very shallow breathing.

After several hours of ventilation on 100 percent oxygen, however, the patient woke. Remarkably, he wasn't groggy or confused, but fully conscious and completely oriented. Yet he had no memory of what happened to him. "All I remember is that I was driving my car back toward town," Altman said. "The next thing I knew, I was waking up here."

The EMT team said they were called to the scene of a one-car accident where Altman's car had run off the road into a ditch. The windshield was broken out, and he was slumped over the steering wheel unconscious.

"Well, we finally know the cause of your illness. Your blood carboxyhemoglobin level is one of the highest the lab has ever seen. You've got carbon monoxide poisoning."

"But why only in the fall and spring?" the chief medical resident wondered aloud. "And why only late in the afternoon?"

The doctors explained their diagnosis, as well as likely sources of carbon monoxide to Altman. They asked him to think back over his daily habits, trying to connect how he might have come in contact with the deadly poison.

He said he bought a used car in March, but hadn't noticed any odors or problems. Typically, he drove with the windows closed when it was cold and open in warm weather. Because he makes so many stops every day, he said he's not really in the car for any length of time until his drive home in the afternoon.

It was those last words that unraveled the mystery. Since Altman's headaches began in March and only occurred in cold weather in the late afternoon, riding for a sustained time with the windows up in a faulty car was the culprit.

Carbon monoxide (CO) is a close chemical gaseous cousin of carbon dioxide (CO2). It is a tasteless and odorless gas and very poisonous. There are thousands of ER visits each year from CO poisoning and several hundred deaths in the U. S. The gas is formed in any heating system where the combustion is partial or incomplete. Home stoves or heating systems not well vented are the most common sources, as are automobiles with improper exhausts or poorly vented engine gases. Home heating systems with no vents are notorious. Charcoal fires inside homes are also sources of fatal carbon monoxide poisoning.

When breathed into the lungs, carbon monoxide quickly combines with hemoglobin and displaces oxygen. As carbon monoxide levels increase, oxygen levels fall. The victim becomes more and more anoxic and, if not removed from the source of the gas, soon dies. Oxygen administration speeds removal of carbon monoxide from its attachment to hemoglobin. Death from the gas is actually an internal asphyxiation, the same as being choked to death.

The fire department was dispatched to find Altman's car. When they tested it for carbon monoxide emissions, they found the levels to be quite high.

Altman had been only minutes away from death, probably saved by the broken windshield that let in fresh air.

Altman had the car repaired and resumed his rounds selling candy and crackers along the back roads. With the exhaust system fixed, he had no recurrence of the poisoning. The case reminds us not only of how dangerous and sneaky carbon monoxide can be, but also that not all seasonal illnesses can be blamed on allergies.

This case was shared by Dr. Jim Jirjis, M.D., M.B.A.

Assistant Chief Medical Officer for Vanderbilt Medical Group
Assistant Professor of Medicine, Vanderbilt University School of Medicine

Chapter Five

Snakes on a Porch *

Dewayne Childs and his wife Edwena bought an old log cabin on the western bank of the Buffalo River. The cabin, built in 1858, was in shambles. But that didn't bother these two. Newly married, young and full of energy, they were excited about restoring it for their first home.

Dewayne had worked as an Emergency Medical Technician (EMT) for the county for more than five years. Before that he worked as a nurse practitioner in a city hospital emergency room. He thought he had seen it all.

A month after moving into the log cabin, Dewayne woke with a severe headache and fever. His temperature was 104 degrees. He hadn't felt well for two days with symptoms he thought were the flu, but this was clearly something else. He told Edwena they needed to get to the emergency room and she needed to drive.

When Dr. Paul Barnett saw Dewayne in the ER, he immediately recognized signs of a serious, even life-threatening infection. Dewayne was "sick out the eyes," a poorly defined term that pediatricians used to describe very sick children. Experienced physicians knew it when they saw it.

There are very few infections that can flatten a healthy person in a few hours. Meningitis would be high on the list. In addition to the severe headache and fever, Dewayne complained of abdominal pain, aching joints and nausea. Soon after he arrived in the ER, he vomited several times.

The physical exam was normal except for the fever and a faint pink rash appearing on the skin of his chest and abdomen. There was no rash on the arms or legs. Barnett thought Dewayne's neck was a bit stiff, enough so to order a spinal tap to check the spinal fluid for meningitis. Without waiting for any lab test results, he started intravenous antibiotics to cover any known infectious organism.

Just after the spinal tap was done, Edwena came into the exam room.

"Dewayne," she said, "did you tell Dr. Barnett about the rats?"

Her sick husband could barely shake his head, "No," he muttered. "You tell him."

Edwena began telling Dr. Barnett a long story that seemed to be going nowhere. One evening at dusk, she said, she was sweeping the front porch of the cabin when she saw what she thought was a limb from a tree. She tried to sweep it off the porch when it started to move. She screamed for Dewayne, and then remembered he wasn't home yet from his shift on the emergency crew.

Dewayne interrupted Edwena. "He doesn't need the whole background. Just the facts."

Edwena continued her story. "When the thing started to move, I knew it was a snake. So I ran to the woodpile and grabbed a big ol' axe. I took it back to the front porch and began choppin' that snake into as many pieces as I could, as fast as I could."

The term "overkill" came to mind as Barnett listened to Edwena's description of how many times she hit that snake. But each time she would lop off a piece, it would squirm a bit. So she kept chopping, determined to be sure that snake — all of it — was dead.

"When Dewayne got home that night, I thought he would be proud of my being so brave," Edwena said. "But he fussed at me! He said it was a rat snake which eats rats, and I shouldn't have killed it. He said it was helping us around that old country cabin. Well, dang it, how was I to know? A snake is a snake."

Sure enough, over the next few weeks the place was overrun with rats. In any given day, they would see at least a half dozen of the nasty rodents running out of the closets, behind the furniture and into the kitchen.

"When Dewayne got sick this morning, he told me it was because of all those rats that come from my killing that snake," she said. "He thinks he's got rat fever, whatever that is."

Dr. Barnett told them he also thought Dewayne had "rat fever," called murine or endemic typhus. He had begun doxyclycline, the antibiotic needed to treat murine typhus. He also used several other antibiotics to cover other possible infections. The spinal fluid was normal, ruling out meningitis. They would have to wait on the test results to know exactly what infection Dewayne had.

Murine typhus is transmitted by the fleas of rats, most frequently in the summer and fall. The infectious organism is classified as a rickettsia. It is difficult to culture, so the diagnosis is confirmed by finding antibodies to the rickettsia in the blood. In this case the suspected organism was rickettsia typhi. The infection can be lethal if not treated.

Several days later, Dewayne's serological test for rickettsia typhi showed a high level of antibodies. The diagnosis of murine typhus was confirmed.

Epidemic typhus, the one responsible for lethal epidemics throughout history in Europe, is transmitted by body lice from person to person. That organism is rickettsia prowasekii. Mortality of epidemic typhus can reach over 50 percent.

The state health department sent a team out to the log cabin and found rickettsia typhi in the feces of the rats. Dewayne had intuitively known what made him sick. The health department instigated a fumigation of the cabin to kill the fleas and put out poisons to kill the rats.

In a few days, Dewayne was much better and ready to go home. He would continue the oral antibiotic for another 10 days. Dr. Barnett wrote out the prescriptions and handed them to Edwena. He asked her to read one of them out loud to her husband:

"No. 1," she began, "Get one black rat snake, two if possible.

"No. 2: Put the snakes under your house.

"No. 3," she paused with a big grin, "Do not kill the snakes."

Case shared by:

Paul Barnett, M.D.
Associate Clinical Professor of Medicine
Department of Medicine
Vanderbilt University School of Medicine.

Chapter Six

*A Lag in Medical Knowledge. ***

Marilyn Potter was rushed to the ER of the local hospital by her fiancé, Boyd Sutterfield. Marilyn had just swallowed all of the pills she had on her bedside table, telling Boyd she hated him and wished to die. She had just celebrated her 29th birthday. The year was early 1977.

In the ER, the team of nurses and Dr. Alex Witherspoon hearing of the suicide attempt rushed to quickly begin IV fluids. They then aspirated and irrigated Marilyn's stomach with saline solutions. Marilyn's blood pressure and pulse were normal. Her breathing appeared normal, as did her blood gases.

Dr. Witherspoon was perplexed by the array of pill bottles brought in with Marilyn. There were all sorts of medications listed on the labels of the empty bottles, including birth control pills, multivitamins, an antihistamine and capsules of vitamin A, vitamin C and Tylenol. What puzzled Witherspoon was the fact none of these pills were thought to be lethal at the time, not even taken all at once as Marilyn claimed she'd done.

Witherspoon began questioning Marilyn about her intent and her state of mind. After several minutes, she began to sob uncontrollably. She told Witherspoon that she wanted Boyd's attention and the only way she knew to get it was to fake suicide. She was careful to use only the pills she thought were safe. She really did not intend to kill herself.

Being extra cautious, the doctor decided to hold Marilyn overnight for observation of her physical and mental states. It was a good call because by the next morning, screening tests showed her liver function was markedly abnormal. Not knowing the cause for this troubling change and concerned for her rapid clinical deterioration, Witherspoon transferred Marilyn to the University Hospital for further evaluation.

By the time of transfer, Marilyn was becoming severely nauseated and vomiting all oral intake. She also was noticeably jaundiced and exhibiting signs of severe liver damage.

The University Hospital had just instituted a clinical pharmacy program. Pharmacists with special training in clinical pharmacology and therapeutics were just beginning to be hired as staff to the larger U.S. hospitals. These new, highly trained pharmacists were now receiving Doctor of Pharmacy (PharmD) degrees. The University Hospital had just engaged Dr. Al Roach as a consulting Clinical Pharmacist. Roach made himself available for any medication or drug problem, be it for information on dosages, interval of administration, potential toxicity, indication, interaction with other drugs, contraindications and other vital information. Soon medical staffs knew to call the clinical pharmacist for any and all medication issues. This new breed of pharmacists changed and improved the face of in-hospital drug administration.

Dr. Roach was called to see Marilyn Potter on her arrival at the University Hospital. The unanswered questions were: If all the drugs she took were not toxic, what was the cause for her deterioration in liver function? Was this due to some combination of the drugs, or was this the result of some drug she hadn't told them she had taken? Most importantly, what could be done to protect or reverse her now failing liver?

Roach, on speaking with Marilyn and her family, determined that the largest dosage of any drug she took was Tylenol in its generic form acetaminophen. A careful search of the usual North American literature revealed no reported toxicity of acetaminophen. Not satisfied, Roach began searching foreign and European literature. It was here he uncovered a drug named paracetamol in the United Kingdom. He quickly discovered it was another generic name for acetaminophen and that the two drugs were identical. What's more, the incidence of liver toxicity for paracetamol was well documented in the European literature.

Now knowing the source of liver damage, Roach found and obtained the known antidote for paracetamol: acetylcysteine whose trade name is Mucomyst. Acetylcysteine acts as a precursor to glutathione, thus helping the body regenerate enough glutathione to prevent further liver damage from the metabolites of acetaminophen (Tylenol).

There are two lessons here: Because none of the existing medical specialties could track all drugs, advanced clinical pharmacists as a new specialty with PharmD degrees provided a necessary — and sometimes critical — piece of the puzzle as newer and more complex drugs were being introduced. Their contribution has greatly enhanced in-hospital care. The perfect example is Marilyn Potter, who may not have survived the liver damage without acetylcysteine discovered by such a pharmacist.

The second lesson, however, lies in the fact that this particular pharmacist wasn't satisfied by his findings in the North American Literature regarding the absence of reported toxicity. Where others might have stopped at this authoritative source, he kept digging. That tenacity most likely saved the patient's life.

Case shared by:

Al Roach, PharmD, FACG
Medical Scientist Director
Ironwood Pharmaceuticals
Nashville, Tennessee

Chapter Seven

*A Dose by Any Other Color... *

Dr. Alan Siegal was finishing his check-out sessions reviewing charts with the medical residents, when Dr. Maxwell Fisher asked him to see one of the clinic patients. Fisher was a second-year resident headed toward a practice of general medicine. Walking down the hall toward the exam room, Fisher quickly briefed Siegal on the case of Jonas Stillman.

Stillman was a 28-year-old mechanic back for a follow-up visit. Dr. Fisher had seen Stillman a month ago and made a diagnosis of hypothyroidism. The patient then had cold intolerance, very dry skin, puffy eyes and poor exercise tolerance. The blood tests had confirmed very low thyroid levels, so Dr. Fisher began Stillman on thyroid replacement therapy with Synthroid , a synthetic thyroid hormone. In the month since Fisher had seen Stillman, all of the symptoms of low thyroid hormone had disappeared. Fisher however said Stillman had a new and unexplained symptom.

When the doctors entered the small exam room, Stillman was sitting on the exam table pulling a towel back and forth across his shoulders. "This itch is killing me," Stillman said. "It's all over, like insects. It won't go away even when I scratch it."

Dr. Siegal examined carefully Stillman's skin and found no lesions or hives. The itching had no visible cause. The patient went on to say how much better he felt on the thyroid replacement generally and he would be well if the itching would quit. "I started to itch about a week after I last saw you," Stillman told Dr. Fisher.

Siegal asked the young resident if he had any idea what might be causing the itch. Fisher said he had no clue.

"What dose of thyroid replacement did you give?" Dr. Siegal continued.

"He is on Synthroid 0.1 milligram daily." Dr. Fisher said. Synthroid is commonly prescribed for hypothyroidism. The dose was about average for replacement.

"Stop the Synthroid 0.1 milligram tablets. Change him to Synthroid 0.05 milligram tablets, two a day," the senior physician said.

Fisher now looked completely puzzled. "But two 0.05 milligram tablets is 0.1 milligram. That's the same dose he's on now."

"I know. Trust me," Dr. Siegal said. "I believe Mr. Stillman's itching will go way."

Fisher wrote a short note in the chart, shaking his head in disbelief. He had no idea what Dr. Siegal was thinking.

When Jonas Stillman returned to see Dr. Fisher a few weeks later, he was a happy man. "Itching went away just like Dr. Siegal said it would."

Fisher was delighted, but still confounded as to how two pills instead of one made a difference, given the same dosage. He rushed to find Dr. Siegal.

Dr. Siegal also smiled at the news and began to explain how he pinpointed the source of the itching.

"I knew 0.1 milligram Synthroid was yellow and I know that the yellow dye in the tablet is Tartrazine," he said. "Tartrazine is also a food coloring with a documented history of occasional allergic reactions. Mustard gets its yellow color from the dye. I recalled another case where Synthroid 0.1 milligram had also caused itching, relieved by using two 0.05 milligram tablets that don't contain the yellow dye. The 0.05 mgm tablets are white."

Dr. Fisher was amazed. "But why don't people get itching from eating mustard?" he asked.

"I suspect they would if they ate it every day and they were susceptible to tartrazine itch, whatever that is. Taking the yellow

Synthroid every day sets up whatever tratrazine dye causes. I don't know the precise allergenic cause for the itch, but it is uncommon.

"In 30 years, this is only the second case I have seen," Dr. Siegel said, "and it's your first, Dr. Fisher. But I bet you will not miss another Synthroid 0.1 tablet itch if you ever see another one."

Case shared by

Dr. Alan Siegal, M.D., M.A.C.P.
Faculty, Medical Education
Baptist Health Systems
Birmingham, Alabama

Chapter Eight

First Diagnosis of Death*

It was my first night on call as a medical intern at Columbia Presbyterian Hospital. I was assigned to cover the private area known as Harkness Pavilion. The year was 1955.

Harkness Pavilion was *the* hospital for the rich and famous of Manhattan and, I suppose, for much of the world at that time. Madam Chiang Kai-Shek, for example, took over an entire floor when she came for her annual checkup. During the year of my internship, the private physicians admitted Elizabeth Taylor, Edward R. Murrow, Rex Harrison and many other celebrities from Broadway, Hollywood and the world of politics. It was one of the main U.S. hospitals for the royal families of Saudi Arabia.

I had lived all my life in the South, went to college and medical school there. New York was a strange territory for me. Southerners were still looked down on as stupid and uneducated. The prejudice was at times palpable. I was a stranger in a very strange land.

Around 2 a.m., I was called to pronounce a patient dead. I jumped out of bed. We slept in our white uniforms, so we were always ready for calls.

After finding my way to the 5th floor, I met the nurse in the dimly lit hallway. She was very official, stern and appeared to be older than my grandmother. Wearing a long white dress with a blue apron and large white nurse's cap, she was from another century.

She looked like I imagined Florence Nightingale might have looked in her later years.

She peered over her glasses as she spoke to me. "Mr. Williams in room 553 quit breathing at 1:54 AM. We need you to pronounce him."[1*]

This being my first official patient, my overriding fear was that I would make a diagnosis of death on a man who was still alive. In some Edgar Allen Poe-like ghoulish scene, I could imagine the poor man waking in horror in the morgue, calling out to some attendant, who would immediately call the chief resident, who would then call the Chairman of Medicine. I shuddered at the thought of being called into his office to be told I that I could not tell a live person from a dead one. I would be banned forever and on my first night as a real doctor.

I had only one thing on my mind when I walked into Mr. William's room: I would not make an overdiagnosis of death. I would make sure he was dead before I said he was dead. I had seen dead patients in medical school, but I had never had to say they were dead. My obsession with making an accurate diagnosis I am sure buried my deeper emotions of facing death. I displaced the thought that here was a person who only a few moments before was an alive human being.

I looked at the chest for several moments. No movement. Then I listened to his heart with my stethoscope for several minutes and at each valve area. No sounds. Then I felt for a pulse at his wrist, then his neck, then for a femoral pulse at his groin. Nothing. No pulse. I actually checked for *rigor mortis*, hoping to find it, but his joints were quite limber.

Then I remembered reading that after death, the arteries in the back of the eye change dramatically. I asked for an ophthalmoscope. While the nurse went for the scope, I went back over each pulse area, listened some more to the heart and even put my ear close to his nostrils, listening for any movement of air. I was becoming more and more confident that Mr. Williams was dead. More confident but still not absolutely sure. No half-dead person was going to get by me and wake up in the morgue.

I looked carefully through the ophthalmoscope and there they were – the small arteries lacing across the retina at the back of the eye with the telltale sign. The red cells had separated from the plasma in alternating dark and clear segments called "boxcars." I knew with certainty that Mr. Williams was dead. His blood had begun to separate.

I turned to the nurse and said, "Mr. Williams is dead."

She looked at me with a dour expression. "Well, aren't you going to pronounce him?"

I was taken completely off guard. What did she mean by "pronounce him?" Here I was in New York City in the inner sanctum of the rich and famous trying to assert myself — and feeling clueless. What strange culture had I landed in? I even wondered if I had missed something in medical school.

I stood up as tall as I could, turned to the nurse, looked at the chart to be sure I had the correct name, and said, "Mr. Jonathan S. Williams is dead."

She didn't budge. "I mean, aren't you going to pronounce him?" Her tone and demeanor were calm like I had omitted some routine step.

Now I was really puzzled. What did she want? What custom or ritual did she mean? Was calling someone dead in New York so different from that in the South? Was this some old world custom?

Finally, I looked around the room to be sure I was alone with the nurse and the dead patient. I then raised my arm and held my hand out over the dead body like some strange priestly ritual and said in my most official voice, "I pronounce Mr. Jonathan S. Williams dead."

With that, the nurse said, "Thank you." She turned and walked out of the room.

I followed her to the nurses' station and entered my note in the chart, carefully documenting all the signs of death I had observed. If somehow Mr. Williams did wake up in the morgue, at least I had made sure I had documented his death.

To this day, I remain mystified by the events of that night. I have never encountered another nurse in more than 50 years who wanted a patient officially pronounced dead. I have told the story to many colleagues, and no one has ever had the same experience or offered a plausible explanation. Was she some strangely religious person? From some obscure cult?

Or worse, in the following years, did she tell her story over and over of the night she got some green intern from the South to actually stick his arm out over a patient and say, "I pronounce this patient dead." I can even imagine her collapsing into laughter as she told the story, repeating the punch line.

Chalk it up to yet another "medical mystery." I will never know the truth about the night I made my first diagnosis of death, nor will I ever forget it.

Story told by Clifton K. Meador, M.D.

Chapter Nine

Medicine Can Be a Humbling Profession *

Ed Clemons had enjoyed a long career as an educator and adminis-trator. Now 58, he had risen to become principal of his local county high school. He also coached the football team as an assistant and taught physics to seniors.

When Dr. Paul Barnett saw Clemons in his office, he found noth-ing of note in the medical history. But his physical examination revealed a large, pulsating mass in the lower abdomen. Barnett or-dered an ultrasound, which showed an aneurysm of the abdominal aorta. An aortic aneurysm is a ballooning and enlargement of the artery leading to the arteries to each leg. This aneurysm measured 8 centimeters in diameter; the normal aorta is around 2 centime-ters in diameter. In other words, the aneurysm was quite large and in danger of rupturing.

A vascular surgeon saw Clemons that day and recommended immediate surgery to repair the aneurysm. If it ruptured, they told him, it would likely be fatal even if he were to get to an emergency room.

But Clemons would have none of it. He refused the surgery, despite all efforts to convince him otherwise. Instead, he asked what symptoms he could expect if the aneurysm ruptured. Barnett described the pain, weakness and nausea and told him to come in immediately if any such symptoms occurred.

A few months went by before Clemons called Barnett. He said he was feeling really bad, pain all over his body, very weak and maybe a bit feverish. Barnett told him to come to the ER immediately.

The vascular surgeon and Barnett met him there. Clemons looked acutely ill, sighing and making slight soft moaning sounds when he exhaled. They did a physical exam, which showed no changes from the months prior. As before, there was no abdominal tenderness. But his temperature was a little over 100, and there was a rash over his legs, arms and abdomen.

Tests were ordered to check on organ function and to re-examine the ultrasound status of the aneurysm. Taking no chances, the team began prepping Clemons for emergency surgery. The one piece of the puzzle that didn't fit was the rash, but because time was of the essence both ignored it and moved forward. "You always have to throw out something," Barnett thought to himself.

As the doctors and staff had been examining and prepping Clemons, an old woman had come into the room quietly several times to clean. She had obviously overheard all of what was going on. Just as Barnett was about to leave the exam room for the last time, she came up to him.

"Excuse me, Doctor," she said gently, "I got 22 grandchildren and dat man got de chicken pox." She pointed at Clemons.

Surely not, Barnett thought, but a good doctor leaves no stone unturned. He went back to look at the rash. She was right. Clemons was about to have complex surgery for the chicken pox.

Barnett says he realized several things in that moment: the need for humility, the importance of remembering that each of us can learn from anyone and that the dismissed symptom can be the key. He thanked the woman and called off the surgery. Clemons recovered uneventfully from the chicken pox.

Clemons returned a month later for an elective repair of his abdominal aneurysm.

Case shared by:

Paul Barnett, M.D.
Associate Clinical Professor of Medicine
Department of Medicine
Vanderbilt University School of Medicine

Chapter Ten

Mysterious Mammaries *

"Herman, you will love this case. It's right down your path," Dr. Steve Stevens said, just returning from the OR after finishing a morning of plastic surgery.

"The man is 38 years old. Has huge breasts. Wants them off. Can you see him?"

Dr. Herman Waring, a consulting endocrinologist, immediately wanted to know more. His role in this case would be to determine why this man's breasts enlarged.

"Look Herman, that's why I am sending him to you," Dr. Stevens interrupted. "I can't sit around asking questions. All I know is his boobs grew over the past few years."

Robert Mac Carter was sitting on the exam table when Dr. Waring came in. Mac Carter was a large man with a dark, full beard. His arms and legs were unusually heavy and hairy. Given this increase in his breast size, Waring immediately began looking for any signs of feminization: a higher pitched voice, feminized hips, loss of body hair. He found none.

In fact, Mac Carter was the opposite of what Waring expected. The man had the size and demeanor of an NFL tight end — big and tough. When he spoke, his answers were simply "yes," "no," or just a few words. It was obvious he did not relish seeing a doctor for this complaint. Waring couldn't help but be struck by the incongruity of this ultra-masculine man with 44D-cup size breasts.

Waring took a long and careful medical history from Mac Carter. There was nothing remarkable in his early life. These days, he was an aeronautical engineer traveling the world as a contractor for several major airlines. He had lived on nearly every continent during the past five years, with most of his time spent in the Philippines.

Yes, he had erections. Yes, he had orgasms. Yes, he had a normal sex drive. Yes, he was heterosexual. No, he had never been married. No, he did not smoke marijuana, which can cause male breasts to grow. None of Mac Carter's actions or body positions were the least bit feminine.

Waring then focused on the endocrine causes for breast growth in a man. Tumors of the adrenals and testicles can secrete estrogens, as can some lung and other cancers. Taking estrogens by mouth will also have this effect. Mac Carter denied taking any medicines at all and, when asked specifically about estrogen tablets, seemed offended. "Of course not," he replied curtly.

Next came the physical examination which revealed large pendulous breasts, at least a D cup. There were no masses. The tissue was quite firm, as sometimes is found in women with unusually large breasts. The chest x-ray showed dense breast tissue with normal lungs. The external genitalia were mature male with no masses felt in the testicles. The remainder of the exam was normal.

Waring ordered all tests measuring estrogen and other hormones controlling sexual development. Results were normal. He thought there had to be some mistake, so he repeated the tests. Again, all normal levels. There was no endocrine explanation for the breast enlargement.

Waring called Dr. Stevens. "Steve, I'm stumped. I have no idea why Mac Carter grew breasts."

"Well, I am taking them off next week," Stevens said. "Will let you know when I get the path report."

The next week, Waring got an urgent call from Stevens. "If you can, get up to the OR. You have got to see this."

Waring prepped quickly, putting scrubs on over his suit. He entered the operating room and stood behind Stevens. When he looked into the open breast tissue, he saw a white substance oozing out onto the surgical drapes.

"What the *hell* is that?' Waring asked.

"It's paraffin," Stevens said. "Very waxy feeling. Both breasts are filled with the stuff."

Both doctors were completely mystified. After the anesthesia wore off, they began to question Mac Carter about how paraffin could have gotten into his breasts. But as before, Mac Carter remained a man of few words. He wasn't talking. The only thing he did say was that he would answer no questions, not now, not ever. No response, no explanation. End of story.

Paraffin injection for breast augmentation was common in the early 20th century but was abandoned because of painful complications. It is still practiced in some Asian countries. Could Mac Carter have been some sort of transgender variant who got breast enlargements with paraffin but then changed his mind? Was there some weird event when he was in Asia that led to the paraffin injections? Neither Stevens nor Waring, even in retrospect, suspected anything unusual about this patient's behavior or demeanor that would lead to such a strange finding.

Two days after surgery, Mac Carter left the hospital. Neither doctor ever saw him again. The mystery was sealed.

Case shared by

Lawrence K. Wolfe, M.D., FACP, FACE
Clinical Professor of Medicine
Division of Diabetes, Endocrinology and Metabolism
Department of Medicine
Vanderbilt University School of Medicine

Chapter Eleven

The eye does not see what the mind is not prepared to know. *

The high school state football championship game was scheduled for the coming weekend between the Black Bears and the Crimson Tigers. Football was big in this Southern state, and excitement was growing. The game would be played on a neutral field in the state's capitol city, about 70 miles from each competing team.

Claude Akin, placekicker for the Black Bears, was warming up during the final practice that Friday. He was getting a feel for the championship stadium's turf and kicking well. After putting a number of balls right through the uprights, however, he was hit by a pain in his lower right leg. It was so sharp, he collapsed to the ground and lay there writhing. It subsided a bit in a few minutes and he managed to get up and walk back to the bench. But no more practice. Something was wrong. The coach told him to ice down the leg below the knee, hoping that would do the trick.

The ice offered temporary relief, but later that afternoon the pain had become so severe that Akin — now crying and moaning continuously — was taken to the ER. The physician there examined it thoroughly, but could find no explanation for the pain.

The teenager couldn't sleep that night, his leg hurt so much. At 3:00 a.m., he woke his parents in the adjoining hotel room and said he had to go back to the ER, but wanted to try a different hospital

43

in hope of answers. By the time the three of them arrived at that ER, Akin was screaming with pain and began to vomit. His parents were anxious and puzzled, given the severity of the pain with absolutely no sign of injury. There was neither redness nor swelling.

The ER physician examined Akin and found no cause for the pain either. A plain x-ray of Claude's leg was normal. All joints in the leg showed full range of motion. The ER physician began to wonder if this could simply be another teenager trying to con drugs, so he asked the Akins if their son was a known user. They were horrified and insulted. They immediately checked their son out of the ER and drove across town to a third ER.

By the time Akin arrived at the third ER, he was prostrate with pain and had to be wheeled inside. Again, the ER physician failed to find a cause and refused to give the young man any narcotic or strong pain medications. He told the parents these extreme "histrionics" coupled with the negative findings suggested malingering and faking.

Angered by the insensitivity of yet another ER physician and frustrated by the failure to get relief, Akin's parents called their family physician back home and described the situation. Dr. Richard Snow had been their family doctor for many years. He had known Claude Akin since childhood — and knew instantly what was wrong with that leg.

"Can only be one thing," he told Akin's father. "He may need immediate surgery. Can you get back here quickly?"

The answer was an unequivocal, "Yes."

"Good," Snow replied. "I'll have Dr. Taylor Wilson, who's an orthopedist, meet you in the ER at St. Paul's."

The Akins rushed the 70 miles back to their hometown hospital. It had been more than 36 hours since the onset of pain in the placekicker's leg. As they drove, their son lay in the back seat, trying in vain to find a position of his body or leg that relieved the excruciating pain.

After Dr. Wilson examined Akin, he said, "This is an anterior compartment syndrome, and we need to do surgery immediately. I am afraid we may be a bit late to save muscle and nerve function in this leg."

The anterior compartment of the lower leg runs down beside the long bone of the shin called the Tibia. The bone, four muscles, nerves, vessels and fascia form a tightly enclosed compartment. Injury to the compartment sets up a vicious cycle of tightly enclosed swelling, occlusion of the veins, compression of the nerves and necrosis (death) of the muscles. All of the factors increase in intensity, eventually leading to death and destruction of all the contents of the tight compartment.

A review of the literature reveals an urgent time window of three to five hours after injury if nerve and muscle function are to be protected. Akin's injury was more than 36 hours old, far too late to save his muscles and nerves. Unfortunately, the young kicker was left with a permanent foot drop and no longer able to play active sports.

The anterior compartment syndrome is relatively rare. Often, its only physical finding is a complaint of severe pain in the leg with little or no visible signs early on. It's one of those diagnoses that must be memorized and remembered in the absence of the common signs of injury like swelling. Only the alert and informed physician will make the diagnosis and see that surgical incisions are made the entire length of the compartment to relieve the swelling and pressure.

In Akin's case, three different ER physicians missed the diagnosis, leading to critical time delays and irreversible muscle and nerve death.

*Case shared by:

Robert Foote, M.D.
Director, Nuclear Cardiology Diagnostic Laboratory
Dartmouth Hitchcock Medical Center
Assistant Professor of Medicine and Radiology
Dartmouth Medical School

Chapter Twelve

A Drug to Prevent a Complication Causes the Complication. *

Jason McKnight had been seeing Dr. Paul Barnett for nearly 10 years. He had adult onset diabetes, now called Type 2.

McKnight was head of a small accounting firm. His compulsive attention to numbers led him to keep meticulous records of his treatment and blood sugar levels, which he measured daily. He also recorded his exercise sessions and his caloric intake and body weight. Nearly all the numbers were very close to normal. The only medicine he was taking was one Metformin tablet daily, which is one of the oral medications for control of blood sugar levels.

Dr. Barnett thought of McKnight as the perfect patient with diabetes. He had never seen anyone take better care of himself. Even McKnight's hemoglobin A1C levels were normal. Hemoglobin A1C is a measure of the average blood sugar level for several months. It is the gold standard for measuring results of treatment in patients with diabetes.

When McKnight called in for an early appointment, Barnett was surprised to hear him describe having symptoms of nerve damage in his legs and feet, called peripheral neuropathy. This is common in many diabetics, but not usually in those who manage their blood sugars as meticulously as McKnight. Examination did, in fact, show a decreased sense of touch and some loss of pain sensation in both feet. Despite excellent management of his blood sugars, McKnight had somehow developed nerve damage.

Nerve damage comes from continued high blood sugars and results from damage to the small blood vessels supplying blood to the nerves in both legs. Tight control of blood sugar usually prevents the damage, but apparently not in McKnight's case. Yet all of his blood tests were again normal, except for a vitamin B12 level that registered at the lower limits of normal.

Dr. Barnett, puzzled by McKnight's developing this complication of diabetes while under good control, referred him to a neurologist, Michael Kaminski. Dr. Kaminski was well known for his diagnostic abilities.

After examining McKnight, Kaminski called Barnett to tell him what he thought might be going on. Kaminski had just read an article describing peripheral neuropathy caused by Metformin, and he referred Barnett to several journal articles.

The articles reported studies of diabetic patients receiving Metformin. Somewhere between 6 and 30 percent of these patients developed low vitamin B12 blood levels. Further studies concluded that Metformin blocks the absorption of vitamin B12 in the intestines. A deficiency of vitamin B12 is usually called pernicious anemia, caused by a lack of absorption of the vitamin. In that sense, the effect of Metformin resembled pernicious anemia.

Kaminski suggested stopping the Metformin and substituting another oral medication for blood sugar control. Within three months, McKnight had a return of normal nerve function to his legs and feet. His vitamin B12 level also returned to normal.

It's a strange coincidence that a medicine aimed at preventing a complication of diabetes should, in fact, create the very complication it was designed to prevent.

This toxic effect of Metformin is something not many doctors know. While the British navy may have known lime juice could prevent scurvy more than 160 years before it was required on all ships, one should hope critical medical information would spread a bit faster in the information age.

Case shared by:

Paul Barnett, M.D.
Associate Clinical Professor of Medicine
Department of Medicine
Vanderbilt University School of Medicine

Chapter Thirteen

*Miss Information**

Boston City Hospital had become so busy for the interns that they had to serve an extra night shift once a week; the "night float" had to be created. The night float intern came on duty at 10 p.m. and worked until 7 a.m., sometimes admitting as many as 10 new patients.

One night, Paul Barnett and a fellow intern were returning from a Celtics basketball game at Boston Garden. They had just seen the great Bob Cousy play and were discussing some of his amazing moves.

They got on the late train heading for Boston City Hospital, both returning for the night float rotation in the ER. The train that time of night was nearly empty. Across the aisle was an old woman who looked homeless. Her hair was unkempt. Her long, stained skirt dragged the floor. She huddled in a ragged coat reading a small book, clutched in filthy hands.

Barnett nudged his friend, "Do you see what she's reading?"

The friend looked for a moment then whispered, "I can't believe it. She's reading a Merck manual."

Merck Manuals were small medical books distributed free to medical students by Merck Pharmaceutical. The book contained short descriptions of nearly all diseases. The idea of a Merck Manual in the hands of a homeless old woman sitting alone on a late night train was so odd, it stuck in Barnett's mind.

Barnett rushed to change into whites and get to the ER before 10 p.m. Just as he came on duty, the resident in charge called out for help with a patient vomiting blood. It was none other than the old woman from the train. The sight of her stopped him in his tracks.

"Get your ass over here and help," the resident yelled. "Don't just stand there."

He watched the woman heaving blood onto the floor and all over her dress. Barnett moved in to help, explaining to the resident how just a few minutes ago he had seen her reading the Merck Manual on the train. The old woman heard him.

Suddenly she stood up and bolted towards the door. As she ran from the emergency room, she spit out several tiny blood-covered balloons, obviously the source of her "vomited" blood.

The resident shouted for the police, ever-present in the ER. They detained her, but it was too late. She had already swallowed the Demerol she had conned out of doctors for her alleged abdominal "ulcer pain."

There simply are no limits to what malingering patients will do to get drugs. We can only wonder what new diseases this woman found in her Merck Manual to serve her devious purposes in subsequent ER visits.

Case shared by

Paul Barnett, M.D.
Associate Clinical Professor of Medicine
Department of Medicine
Vanderbilt University School of Medicine

Chapter Fourteen

An Uncommon Cure *

Walter McKenzie was a patient of old Dr. Smithers for over 2 decades. When it was time for Smithers to retire, he referred McKenzie to Dr. Jim Jirjis, a young internist. By this time, McKenzie was 78 years old.

On his first visit to see the new doctor, McKenzie brought a stack of his old medical charts several inches thick. The two met and talked for a few minutes, then Jirjis told McKenzie he would review the records and see him for a complete examination the following week. As was his practice, Jirjis read every page and reviewed all the lab work for the past 23 years that Dr. Smithers had cared for McKenzie.

Jirjis was impressed with the meticulous notes old Dr. Smithers kept. He easily followed the life history and clinical course of first a man in robust health, then married, having two sons and finally moving on through the middle years to his current senior age. Many years ago, McKenzie had developed Type 2 Diabetes. Dr. Smithers's notes describe a slow progression of various unrelated illnesses: pneumonia with flu, an inguinal hernia operation and a fracture of the wrist from a fall. The diabetes, as is common, worsened over the years, requiring diet, exercise, oral diabetes pills and, ultimately, when the pills were maximized and no longer sufficient, the addition of insulin.

As unremarkable as the charts' information was overall, one thing caught Dr. Jirjis' attention: He began to notice in the chart a slow and gradual trend of the fasting blood sugar levels decreasing over the years. In the early years, the levels seemed to average nearly 250 mgm%. In those days, a normal blood sugar was considered to be less than 140.

When the test for hemoglobin A1C levels became available, McKenzie's were also quite high. Hemoglobin A1C levels measure blood sugars attached to hemoglobin and give a measure of the average blood sugar levels for the previous several months. It is now the gold-standard measurement of diabetic control.

Despite these high numbers early on, Dr. Jirjis noted on McKenzie's first visit with him that the patient was off all of his medications, including the pills and the insulin. Yet, inexplicably, his blood sugars were completely normal at around 100. The hemoglobin A1C level was also normal at 6.5%.

What had at one point been severe, advanced diabetes had gradually gone away without a trace and while receiving no medication or insulin.

When Dr. Jirjis asked McKenzie about this dramatic turn of events, he simply said, "Old Doc Smithers, I guess, cured my diabetes."

At first Jirjis couldn't believe he had witnessed a complete cure of diabetes. No colleague had ever seen such a case. Dr. Jirjis was totally perplexed.

In the months after that initial enigmatic meeting with Dr. Jirjis, McKenzie began to have episodes of emotional irritation, becoming very irritable with no cause. Later the episodes were followed by loss of consciousness. The first time occurred in church when he fell to the floor in the middle of a hymn. These symptoms were all consistent with low blood sugar.

Jirjis immediately knew there was only one possibility: McKenzie's body was somehow being exposed to insulin. The patient was either injecting himself with insulin and not telling anyone, or he was making insulin from his pancreas.

He quickly ruled out surreptitious insulin and honed in on the pancreas. How could a pancreas that made too little insulin suddenly switch to making too much?

Dr. Jirjis ordered tests, among them a CT scan of McKenzie's abdomen. It revealed the answer: a malignant tumor of the pancreas known as an insulinoma. The cancer had already spread to the liver. McKenzie lived only a few more months, dying in protracted hypoglycemia and coma from the malignant insulinoma of his pancreas.

How strange can nature get? Tissues once deficient in producing insulin became malignant, secreting excessive amounts – a weird irony of biology.

Malignant pancreatic tumors secreting insulin are quite rare, occurring in about four per million person years. Even more rare is the coexistence of an insulinoma occurring in a patient with diabetes mellitus. Only a few cases have been reported. (See Chapter notes.)

Further compounding the uniqueness of this amazing case is the fact that Dr. Jirjis's first meeting with McKenzie happened to perfectly coincide with his pancreas making exactly the right amount of insulin to "treat" his diabetes. The coincidence is remarkable.

Case shared by:

Jim Jirjis, M.D., MBA
Assistant Chief Medical Officer for Vanderbilt Medical Group
Assistant Professor of Medicine
Department of Medicine
Vanderbilt University School of Medicine.

Chapter Fifteen

Shining a Light on the Problem *

The hospital was nothing new to Gertrude Amarill. She had been an emergency room nurse for seven years. Being a patient, however, was something that had become all too common recently. On this day, she, a 32-year-old woman, was being admitted to the Regional Medical Center for recurring breast masses. This was her 13th admission.

Peter Seinfold was the admitting surgical resident. In his admission history and physical exam write-up of Ms. Amarill, Dr. Seinfold recorded the recurring admissions and failures of therapy. The exact nature of the recurring left breast masses had not been consistently defined. Numerous biopsies had been taken. Most were read as "nonspecific inflammatory reaction. Rule out deep fungus infection." Several were read as "suspicious of unusual form of breast cancer." Still others were read as "multiple breast abscesses, infecting organism unknown."

On her last admission, a partial resection of the left breast was performed. Several areas of chronic inflammation were seen microscopically. In addition, there were two small acute abscesses. Cultures revealed two infecting bacterial organisms: staph aureus and E. Coli, suspicious of fecal or other contamination. Examination of the breast prior to surgery revealed extensive scarring and depressed areas. The overall size of the affected left breast was at least half the size of the healthy right breast.

Repeated questions to Ms. Amarill revealed no clues. She denied all forms of digital or oral manipulation by herself or other people. She also denied traveling anywhere out of the ordinary or having contact with unusual animals. She kept no pets in her apartment.

Most physicians who saw her suspected some sort of self-infliction or infliction by someone else. She denied all these accusations. She insisted the lesions occurred spontaneously every month or so. There was no seasonal pattern to their appearance; she had been admitted in as many summer months as winter months.

Dr. Seinfold was determined to pin down an etiology for the breast lesions, which he strongly suspected were self-inflicted. He developed the idea of applying a tracer solution to the surgical dressing. He soaked a new dressing in the tracer solution and applied it to the left breast.

After some research, Seinfold had decided on fluorescein which shows up under ultraviolet (UV) light. It's used in ophthalmology to scan the cornea for abrasions. It's also used in lifeboats and life vests to help find those lost at sea. The fluorescein is released into the water and the fluorescence can then be seen from the air by search planes. The attending surgeon agreed to the fluorescein test.

Dr. Seinfold applied the harmless chemical to the dressing and skin of Ms. Amarill's left breast without telling her. All along, she insisted she had not, nor would she ever, touch the dressing or any area of the breast. Whether or not she was telling the truth would be revealed.

On her next clinic visit, an UV light was shone on her hands. Both glowed brightly fluorescent. Despite continuing to deny the obvious, she was persuaded to admit herself to the psychiatric inpatient unit for an extended stay.

Under psychiatric care, Ms. Amarill finally admitted to harming her breast. She had used her own fecal material as the infecting agent. No reason or motivation was ever uncovered, and after a month's stay in the unit she was released. She eventually moved to another town. There was no way to determine the eventual outcome of her breast lesions.

As noted in Chapter 3. (the woman who cut her gums to produce a bloody sputum), there are four general forms of self-harm:

Munchausen Syndrome where the patient moves from hospital to hospital with the intent of being dramatic with self-inflicted disorders; Munchausen by proxy where another person secretly inflicts harm on another person, usually a mother on a child; self-harm for a tangible gain, such as getting illicit drugs or work compensation; and self-harm with no tangible gain, apparently for some unmet personal gain. This is called a factitious disorder

Gertrude Amarill fit the last category. She had no tangible gain from her abscesses. Some unknown, deep psychiatric disturbance drove her to do what she did to herself. As is the case for many such patients, she was lost to follow-up, but hopefully not to further psychiatric care.

This case was shared by a colleague who wishes to remain anonymous.

Chapter Sixteen

What You Don't Know Can Kill You *

Matt Graton was a cotton farmer in West Tennessee, living on the banks of the Tennessee River about a hundred miles from Nashville. Graton had turned 56 in late August, just before cotton picking time.

Graton had enjoyed unusually good health with no serious illnesses. That's why he was surprised to wake one morning with severe shaking chills. His wife, Mabice, took his temperature: 104 degrees. This was serious, so they headed for the hospital in Nashville. By the time they arrived, a red rash covered his arms and legs.

After Graton's admission to the hospital, the medical housestaff began the workup to identify the cause for the fever. Under the supervision of Dr. Robert Latham, blood and urine cultures were collected, along with complete blood count and chemistry screening tests. All tests were normal, except for a very low platelet count. Platelets are essential for clotting, seen as small particles circulating in the blood. Bleeding occurs when the platelet count is low, explaining the hemorrhagic rash seen on Graton.

Anyone with sudden fever and rash coming in the summer in Tennessee should be suspected of having one of the tick-transmitted infections. The most common one in Tennessee is Rocky

Mountain spotted fever, caused by ticks that attach to deer, possums and other wild animals.

When asked if he had gotten any tick bites, Graton answered, "Why, hell yes I get ticks. You can't farm and not get some ticks."

That answer was enough for Latham to begin full antibiotic coverage for Rocky Mountain spotted fever. Within three days, Graton's temperature and platelet count returned to normal and he was pleading to get home for cotton picking. He was discharged to finish a full two weeks of Doxycycline antibiotic.

A few days after Graton went home, test results on the blood mailed off to a special lab for tick testing showed no antibodies for any of the tick-borne diseases. Dr. Latham scratched his head. Graton had all of the symptoms of Rocky Mountain spotted fever; he had recent tick bites; summer was the right time of year for ticks; and the fever and platelets returned to normal with antibiotic treatment. If Graton didn't have Rocky Mountain spotted fever, he must have something very much like it. Latham filed the case in his mental file of strange and puzzling patients.

In late November, Dr. Latham got a long distance call from Matt Graton. Graton said he woke with severe chills and fever and, again, a slight rash.

"Can't be no ticks this time," Graton said. "We've had some hard freezes and I been inside for about a week. I'm heading your way for treatment."

Again Graton was admitted to the hospital and again the work-up was negative except for the low platelet count and fever. Despite the highly unlikely possibility of a tick being the culprit, Graton's blood was sent for study of Rocky Mountain spotted fever and all the other tick-borne infections. In addition, blood was frozen and held for future studies if needed. All the antibiotics given on the August admission were again used. In a few days, the fever and platelet count returned to normal and Graton was discharged to home.

As expected, the test results for tick-borne infections again returned as negative. Latham was even more puzzled and this time signed out Graton as "fever and thrombocytopenia (low platelets) of unknown origin."

In early January, Graton was admitted again with the identical story and findings: high fever and low platelets. Latham was convinced they were missing something obvious. He spent several hours with Graton and his wife tracing a full day in their lives: where they went, where they shopped, what they ate and drank, what pets lived in the house and the state of those pets' health, and on and on down a long list of environmental exposures and possible toxins. Nothing seemed to explain the recurring illness. As before, the antibiotics appeared to work and Graton went back home.

Two months later, Graton showed up in the emergency room, having called Dr. Latham to say he was on his way with the same symptoms. When Latham arrived in the ER and found Graton's exam room, the patient had some news.

"You know, Doc," he said, "I think I may have the answer."

Graton went on to explain how he sometimes got severe leg cramps at night. He kept a bottle of Quinine capsules on his bedside table and took a capsule whenever these cramps occurred. He had been using it safely for years.

"But you got me to thinking with all those questions last time," he continued. "I thought back over the time in August, and then in November, then in January when I got sick. And then I recalled that those are the only times I had to take my quinine for cramps. I had bad cramps last night and took my quinine and here I am sick again."

Latham nodded knowingly, relieved to finally have an answer to the mysterious fever and rash.

Reactions to quinine are many and varied, including renal failure, severe clotting, liver toxicity and neurological damage, in addition to fever and low platelets.[1] Since quinine for leg cramps is usually taken infrequently, it can be difficult to associate with an acute illness. Because Graton had taken it safely for so long, he had no reason to consider it toxic. But over time, he had developed a dangerous sensitivity.

This case shows how vital information can sometimes be buried in our memory, unavailable to recall. It was only on the fourth episode of chills, fever and low platelets that Graton thought of the quinine. The extensive questioning by Dr. Latham had prompted

Graton to think of all possible causes, finally surfacing the quinine from deep memory.

In any patient like Graton, the number of possible offending agents is infinite. No list of possible toxic agents could ever cover all possibilities. Therefore, it is essential to enlist the patient in the search, as this case illustrates.

*Case shared by

Robert H. Latham, M.D.
Chief of Medicine & Chief of Infectious Diseases
St. Thomas Hospital
Nashville, Tennessee

Chapter Seventeen

Out of the Mouths of Babes *

When Curt Tribble was 12 years old, he often went on calls with his dad, the senior Dr. Tribble. His father, a surgeon, was director of the trauma service at the largest hospital in the city.

One night a call came from the ER saying that an elderly woman sitting on her porch had been shot several times with stray bullets. Young Curt raced with his father to the ER.

They were surprised to find the woman conscious, alert and with stable vital signs. By the ripped places in her clothing, they counted what appeared to be six bullet holes in the clothing. The fact that she was stable puzzled Dr. Tribble. He expected shock or at least a high pulse rate and/or a low blood pressure, but both measurements were normal.

He began examining the patient for bullet wounds, but — what's this? — there were none. He ordered x-rays of her chest and abdomen, looking for bullets or areas of trauma. When the films were put up, again there were no bullets visible anywhere in her body. Exploratory surgery was the next consideration.

Young Curt, now thoroughly engaged in the puzzle, piped up, "Maybe the bullets passed under the loose folds of skin, like between her right breast and her abdomen."

His father turned to him, "Now how on earth could <u>that</u> happen, smart alec?!?"

"Well, we heard she was on the porch," the boy reasoned. "Maybe she heard the gunfire and bent over and the bullets passed in and out of the parts of her that were hanging down and then went on between her legs and ended up in the front of the house behind."

The group of doctors looked at one another, thinking. Maybe their "smart alec" young friend just might be right. They decided someone should call a witness to the shooting for more details on exactly what happened.

Sure enough, the witness confirmed the boy's theory. When the woman bent over, the bullets had passed through her clothing but not into her body. Surgery was cancelled, and the woman was discharged the next day in good shape.

A good surgeon must know when and when not to operate, something Curt Tribble learned at an early age. It's no surprise that this astute young fellow followed his father's footsteps into medicine. Today, he is a renowned surgeon.

Case shared by:

Curt Tribble, MD
Professor of Surgery
Chief, Division of Cardiothoracic Surgery
Vice Chair, Department of Surgery
Medical Director of Transplantation
University of Mississippi

Chapter Eighteen

Keeping Secrets *

I was a second year medical resident in New York City at Columbia Presbyterian Hospital. It was late summer of 1956.

I turned the corner of the ward entrance and ran into Dr. Claude Hornsby, one of my attending physicians. He said, "I've been looking for you to ask a favor."

He went into some detail about his serving as the company physician for a large manufacturing company. Many physicians in those days had such "retainer" contracts, making themselves available to be on call to treat the senior executives whenever needed. He then told me there was an upcoming convention in San Juan, Puerto Rico, he was supposed to attend but couldn't. The company wanted an American physician with the group at all times. In need of a substitute, he wondered if my wife and I could get away and serve as the convention doctor in his place.

This sounded like heaven to me. A free trip and vacation! I raced to the office of my chief and, to my surprise, got his permission to be off duty for two weeks.

We would be staying at the Caribe Hilton in the full lap of luxury. I would have no assigned duties, only to be available 24 hours a day for the entire week of the convention. We had all sorts of group activities to join: deep sea marlin fishing, golfing, sightseeing around the old town of San Juan and mostly sitting around the hotel pool, basking in the sun. What a difference from hospital duties in New York.

I got to know most of the executives of the company and enjoyed hearing their life stories and experiences. Most started drinking in the morning and were sauced by late afternoon. Since I was on medical call, I declined any drinking in case I was needed. There was a dinner and entertainment every night.

On the last night of the convention, there was a special dinner with formal dress. Thus far, I had not been called to see a single patient. But just before dinner, I got a call from one of the conventioneers.

"Can you come check on my roommate? I think he's just drunk. He's been passed out. I just want to be sure he's OK."

I said I would be right there and left the banquet hall headed towards the hotel room.

The caller opened the door and led me to the couch where the man was passed out. He thanked me for coming and left to go to the banquet, leaving me alone with the stuporous man.

I brought my black bag, so I took the man's blood pressure and pulse. Both normal. He was mumbling a bit, so I asked him several questions. All he ever said that I understood was, "Ok. Just need sleep. Leave alone."

I pondered the situation carefully. Here was a man, obviously drunk and passed out. But what if it were not that simple? What if he had some serious disease masked by this drunken state — say, meningitis or some stroke or maybe heart failure or sepsis and on and on down a long list of possibilities. I tried to do a neurological exam, but the man was limp. I did get him to stick out his tongue and move his eyes in all directions. His reflexes were all present. He felt pain when I pinched him.

I thought back to the year before when I had to pronounce a man dead and was so worried about making a false diagnosis of death. Missing a diagnosis of death would pale beside missing a serious disease in a living person, especially since this was my one case during the entire week. The only reason I was at the convention was to safeguard the executives.

I sat there for several minutes wondering what to do. I hadn't done anything all week and thought I should at least do something beyond just checking the man out. I remembered scenes from movies in which drunks were given coffee to bring them around. So I ordered coffee from room service and waited, listening to the man make deep snoring sounds. I kept going over and over what I might have missed.

When the coffee came, I poured a cup and offered it to the man. I propped him into a sitting position and spooned a few sips into this mouth. I added a touch of sugar, thinking it might taste better. Eventually, I managed to get most of the coffee down him between his mumbling, "OK, OK. I'm fine. Need sleep."

Out of ideas at this point, I stretched him out on the sofa and covered him with a blanket, left the room and returned to the banquet to find my wife. I told her what had happened.

About 15 minutes later, my name came over the loudspeaker system. I was to find the nearest phone to take a call.

"Are you the one who was just in my room?" the voice on the phone asked.

I said I was just in room 413.

"Well that's my room. I'm Charlie Johnson. Thank you so much. The coffee and sugar you added jarred me into consciousness just enough to take my sugar pill. I am a diabetic on insulin, and I was having a severe insulin reaction. Stupid me, I didn't eat lunch. But I'm fine now, thanks to you. You saved my life."

I was so taken back I didn't know what to say.

"Oh, by the way," he continued. "You have to swear you will tell no one that I am diabetic. I would get fired if anyone in the company found out. They do not tolerate any chronic illnesses."

I tried to convince him he should tell his boss, that there could be another life-or-death situation and people around him should know what to do. Still, he refused. He said he would hold me to my word not to tell anyone — ever.

In a few minutes, Johnson appeared in the banquet hall and roamed table to table. He was clearly one of the most popular men at the convention, and everyone had heard about his drunken state. His roommate had told everyone that Johnson was passed out and how he had summoned me to make a "house call" for his inebriated friend. Each table burst into laughter as Johnson approached, completely surprised to see him conscious and so full of life. He kept pointing over at me each time as if to say, "He's the one that did it. Best drunk doctor I know. "

Johnson eventually made his way to my table, stuck out his hand and slapped me on the back. He laughed and gave me a big wink. "You sure know how to make coffee," was all he said.

All through the banquet, many of the men came up to me, most wanting to know what I gave Johnson. "What in hell did you put in that coffee?" Or, "I want some of that." Or, "You are really one hangover doctor." And on and on. Each time I felt a mixture of feelings, mostly the suppressed urge to tell people what really happened.

From time to time in the passing years, I reflect on the events of that evening. I kept my vow to hide Johnson's secret and told no one until now. It has been 56 years. I think I can safely assume Johnson is dead.

I cannot make any deep meanings out of the evening. But I am still in awe over how the happenstances worked to save Johnson's life. Here I was on a paid vacation to luxury, a second-year resident in medicine, called to see an unconscious man. By luck only, I added sugar to coffee, only because I liked sugar in my own coffee, not because I thought of diabetes or hypoglycemia or any of that. I had missed the one condition I should have considered. Even for physicians — young ones like me, as well as the most educated and practiced ones — blind luck sometimes operates out of nowhere.

Story told by Dr. Clifton Meador

Chapter Nineteen

2+2=Fortunate *

Carl Simons came home around lunch time and began cooking hamburgers.

Within an hour, the young man developed a severe headache, nausea and vomiting. He had a friend take him to the ER, where he was admitted with a suspected cerebral hemorrhage.

CT scan of the brain was normal, but he was admitted for observation and further studies. Simons, 28, mentioned to the admitting resident Dr. Clark Brown that, ironically, his roommate had also been admitted to the hospital's Intensive Care Unit (ICU) that morning. A neighbor had seen the ambulance and called the hospital to check on him. Simons didn't have any more details, because he had been working at his job at the time. Dr. Brown listened, but was mostly focused on his frustration over not being able to make a definitive diagnosis on Simons.

That evening, the Chairman of the Department of Medicine scheduled the first monthly orientation sessions for new housestaff. Attendance was mandatory. Conversations soon turned to which resident had the most interesting case. Dr. Blair Wiggins, a resident rotating on the Intensive Care Unit, told the story of a truck driver named Steve Rogers, age 29, who had been admitted to ICU that day from the ER. Initially, Rogers was unconscious and completely unresponsive. After intubation, he was placed on a ventilator. All blood gases and other studies were normal. As Dr. Wiggins was signing out to come to the orientation, however, the patient had begun to move his arms a bit. Wiggins said no one involved in the case had any idea what had caused Rogers to stop breathing.

Clark Brown, also at the meeting, began talking to Wiggins about other patient histories from the week. Brown was telling Wiggins about a frustrating case in the ER, a guy named Carl Simons, whom he couldn't diagnose. Suddenly, Brown remembered what Simons had said about his roommate and told Wiggins. Rogers must be Simons roommate!

Wait a minute. Two roommates. Sick on the same day. Both with undiagnosed illnesses, one near fatal. The two residents immediately came to the same conclusion: There must be something toxic in the apartment.

Wiggins called the resident covering for him in the ICU. "I think we know what's wrong with Steve Rogers. Get a carboxyhemoglobin stat!" He related Dr. Brown's story of the roommate being admitted the same day. "And get one on Carl Simons down on 6-C, too."

The carboxyhemglobin level on Rogers came back very high, proving carbon monoxide poisoning. The level on Simons was also high but significantly lower than Rogers', indicating exposure to the poisonous gas but not as much.

The fire department was notified, and the young men's apartment was inspected. Fire inspectors traced the source of the carbon monoxide to a second hand unventilated stovetop cooker the duo had purchased.

When Steve Rogers recovered, he told his story. He had come home from work and started cooking supper, but quickly developed a severe headache and nausea. He decided to lie down and rest but became sicker and sicker. Fortunately, he was able to crawl to the phone and call 911. When the EMT arrived, he was unconscious. They rushed him to the ER on 100% oxygen by mask.

Carbon monoxide is a gas that comes from incompletely combusted fuel. It's odorless and tasteless. Most often it comes from poorly ventilated cooking equipment in homes or from exhaust fumes in automobiles. The gas binds tightly to hemoglobin, preventing oxygen from binding. The result is a very low level of oxygen in the blood. The victim can die from anoxia. The carbon monoxide can be displaced by breathing 100 percent oxygen. (As described in Chapter 4. Seasonal Disorder)

The perplexing thing about carbon monoxide poisoning is that the routine blood gas measurements are all normal even in the face of high levels of carboxyhemoglobin. Partial pressure of oxygen (P02) is normal. Physicians must think of carbon monoxide and order a specific test to measure the level.

This case was the confluence of several remarkable coincidences. Because both men wound up in the same hospital and the conscious roommate happened to mention his unconscious roommate, the two residents at the same housestaff meeting put the puzzle together. Both young men recovered. They did not, however, keep the cooker.

***This case was shared by**

Jim Jirjis, M.D., M.B.A.
Assistant Chief Medical Officer for Vanderbilt Medical Group
Assistant Professor of Medicine
Department of Medicine, Vanderbilt University School of Medicine.

Chapter Twenty

A Korean Experience *

Dr. John Newman had just completed his medical residency in 1974 when he was called to active duty in the U.S. Army Medical Corps. His assignment was to be in South Korea as an internist in Mobile Army Surgical Hospital (MASH) Unit #43, located 20 miles from the Demilitarized Zone (DMZ) near the town of Uijongbu, about 10 miles north of Seoul. This was the last functioning MASH unit that descended from the Korean war, which ended in 1953. Many of the M*A*S*H episodes on TV were based on stories from this unit.

During his tour of duty, Newman had seen an accumulation of diseases that were almost never seen in their natural state in the U.S. He saw many rare cases, including raging hyperthyroidism in a young woman that had gone untreated for a year, blue baby syndrome in a teenage boy, all manner of intestinal parasites and advanced tuberculosis. He was struck by the power of Western medicine to treat these diseases.

One day during his last week of duty before leaving the country, Newman had finished sick call and was back in his hooch organizing and packing his belongings. He got a call from the ER that a farm woman wanted him to look at her daughter.

The Korean assistant calling Dr. Newman seemed overwhelmed by the intensity of the mother. She pleaded, "I think you should see, Captain Newman. Mother carry daughter. Cannot walk."

Newman thought the patient might be a baby or child whose care would be outside his training in adult medicine. Still, he volunteered, "Have her bring the child to my hooch."

The Korean assistant led the way, ushering a withered, stooped country woman in her 40s. She wore multiple layers of cotton clothing, plastic sandals and saggy wool socks. They entered Newman's hooch. "Mother name Eon Gangnam Kim," the assistant said. "Daughter name Su Na Kim."

Eon Gangnam Kim's face was ruddy brown and leathery from working outside in the sun and cold for many years. On her back was a teenage girl as big as she was. The girl rode piggyback, clinging to her mother's neck and shoulders. The older woman walked in a shuffle, not lifting her feet, but carrying the weight strongly.

Newman's first thought was that this was a congenital disorder or cerebral palsy, but the girl had normal attention and looked very anxious and tearful.

"How long Su Na no walk?" Newman lapsed into the pigeon English so common to Americans when talking to non-English speakers.

"Five week." the Korean assistant interpreted. "Many Korean doctors, no help."

Newman became intrigued, realizing the problem was recent, still acute.

Newman had the mother unload the girl on his bed and examined her. She could not move her legs voluntarily. They were slightly stiff, but when he struck her patellar tendon with the rubber hammer the girl's leg shot out and went into spasm.

Newman was stunned, since he had expected little or no reflexes. But he recognized these symptoms: The girl had spastic paraparesis of both legs. He had read about it, but never seen a case. This type of paralysis occurs when a spinal tumor blocks brain impulses to the legs but preserves lower neurological reflex arcs. The Korean assistant undressed the girl, revealing the problem: a large grapefruit-sized tumor under the skin on her spine in the center of her upper back.

Newman knew of a neurosurgeon assigned to the 121st Hospital in Seoul, the major Army Hospital in Korea. He spoke to him on the phone. Newman thought the girl had either a spinal tumor or a rare complication of spinal tuberculosis, called Pott's disease. In Pott's disease, the tuberculosis grows in the spinal disc and expands into the bone and compresses the spinal cord, mimicking a cancer. The neurosurgeon doubted Newman's story but agreed to take the case. The MASH ambulance crew drove her down to the Yongsan base in Seoul.

As Newman was about to leave the MASH a few days later, he got a message that the girl's problem was indeed tuberculosis and the infection had been decompressed surgically. The young girl was already getting partial recovery of her leg function.

Dr. Newman was struck by seeing something that existed only in textbooks in the States. By simple application of modern surgery plus antibiotics, they had saved and preserved the girl's life — all thanks to a rubber hammer and a telephone call to the right doctor who knew how to use a scalpel around the spine. Remarkably, there were no CT or MRI scans, no labs, no computer notes, no consent forms, no liability risk, no HIPPA protection of insurability, no billing, no contracts, no consultants and no anxious hospital administrators.

As Dr. Newman boarded the helicopter headed back to Japan and the real world, he wondered if he would ever have so much fun and impact on people's lives as he had during his tour of duty at the 43rd MASH unit in Korea.

*** Case shared by:*

John Newman, M.D.
Elsa S. Hanigan Professor of Pulmonary Medicine
Division of Pulmonary and Critical Care Medicine
Vanderbilt University School of Medicine

Chapter Twenty One

Gut Reaction *

Sheldon Smaldon, a 40-year-old executive, suffered from chronic and persistent anxiety since early childhood. For the past three years, he had frequent panic attacks so severe he finally stopped driving. Public transportation was his only means of travel. He did, however, manage to keep working at a billing and accounting firm.

Dr. Simon Sedon, a psychiatrist, started seeing and treating Smaldon. Over the past three years, he found Smaldon to be obsessed with self-doubt and negative thinking. On some visits, Smaldon went over and over the same issues. He seemed stuck in certain ruminations and patterns of thought.

Sedon used cognitive therapy to treat Smaldon for generalized anxiety disorder. He also prescribed Celexa 10 mgm daily and Xanax on a limited, as-needed basis. On this program, the doctor estimated Smaldon had a 50% reduction in symptoms.

In 2005, Dr. Sedon took a yearlong sabbatical, transferring Smaldon's care to a colleague. When Sedon returned, he was surprised to run into Smaldon at a social gathering. He was even more surprised when Smaldon told him he had been cured of his panic attacks and anxiety. He had been able to commit to his girlfriend and they had married, which signaled a huge step forward in his recovery. His wife was now pregnant with their first child, he said. Smaldon then thanked Dr. Sedon for his previous and compassionate care.

Completely puzzled and taken back by this miraculous recovery, Sedon asked Smaldon how he thought this cure came about.

Smaldon said he had read about how anxiety can be associated with Celiac disease. Celiac disease is caused by sensitivity to gluten, a principal ingredient of wheat. Smaldon had himself tested and found he was, in fact, sensitive to gluten. Armed with this new information, he began avoiding all products containing gluten and found his anxiety diminished.

In a few months of this regime, he had recovered completely. He could now concentrate on his spiritual meditations, something he couldn't do before. His fear of commitment had also dissolved, and he proposed marriage. Now, with the baby on the way, life was good.

Smaldon again thanked Sedon for his care and said he just wanted to be sure the doctor knew about gluten sensitivity and its association with anxiety. This was the first time Sedon had ever heard of the connection, he confessed. He thanked Smaldon for sharing the information.

The exact biochemical mechanism between gluten sensitivity and altered brain function and anxiety is unknown, but the relationship has been clearly established from clinical studies. Gluten testing will likely become another avenue for psychiatrists seeking answers to patients' anxiety.

This case also demonstrates how sometimes the one with the most at stake — the patient — can become their own best sleuth. That said, with so much medical information and misinformation available on the internet today, doctors worry about patients self-diagnosing, doing real harm or, at the very least, scaring themselves needlessly. But, when explored discerningly, some of the information out there can also prove helpful. Smaldon, who at last report remained free of his anxiety, is proof of that.

*Case shared by:

Will Van Derveer, M.D.
Private Practice of Psychiatry
Boulder, Colorado

Chapter Twenty Two

Bite the Hand That Feeds You *

Cecil Norman was a character. A veteran of World War II, he served as an infantry soldier in the Battle of the Bulge where he was wounded in combat. His left leg was hit by shrapnel, but he recovered with no lasting limitations.

Since the war, Norman lived on a small farm in the poorest county in Georgia. He, his third wife and her mother shared a double-wide trailer on the rugged northeast Georgia land. He did odd jobs and barely eked out a living.

Norman had noticed a weakness in both legs that was getting worse, as well as a tingling, odd kind of pain in both feet. Walking was becoming more difficult. He wondered if the old war wound was acting up, so he sought medical care at the Veterans Administration Hospital.

The medical team at the VA Hospital was well defined. For each 20-bed ward, there were two interns, a medical resident and an attending senior physician. Paul Barnett was the attending physician on Norman's ward. Dr. Barnett was in private practice of internal medicine and, like many private doctors, volunteered as an attending physician for a month, rounding three times a week.

Cecil Norman tried to get up from his chair when the team of doctors approached his bed area, but he couldn't. He described in detail how his problem had begun with just the tingling. Then he said his legs got weak, and now he was having trouble even walking.

"Hell, I don't want to be no cripple," he said in a voice loud enough to entertain the other 19 patients on the open ward, "Not what you call a '*parapleeg*' or whatever."

The team listened carefully, laughing with Norman's little jokes. He was clearly enjoying himself. Soon the whole ward was laughing, joining in the act.

Norman settled into the slow and measured pace of the workup process in the VA system. By the end of the first week, the blood work results were finally back. One of the interns on Norman's case, Dr. Tom McElroy, reviewed them. In addition to the routine tests, McElroy had ordered vitamin B12 levels and some other measures that might point to the cause of Norman's peripheral neuropathy. All tests were normal, which meant that the nerves to his legs were injured from some unknown cause.

Another week passed waiting on some other tests and a consultation with the neurologist. At the end of that week, Dr. Barnett, Dr. McElroy and the other interns entered the ward to check on their patients. Much to their surprise, Norman was standing by his bed.

"Hello, Doc!" Norman began. "I'm just sittin' here doing nothin' and gettin' well at the same time. Just look at me walk now! Hell, I think I could run some if I had to." Norman proceeded to strut up and down the length of the ward, saluting the other patients.

The team immediately examined him and found the signs of nerve damage were now much less. The feeling had returned to his feet.

"Doc, ain't no sense in my sittin' in this here hospital gettin' well. Hell, I can do that at home," Norman announced. "Besides, I can get me some beer and enjoy life there. I'm goin' home this afternoon."

His doctors tried to talk him out of leaving, but Norman insisted he was fine. That afternoon, he signed himself out AMA (against medical advice).

Three weeks later, Norman showed up in the emergency room in a wheelchair. Dr. McElroy saw him the next morning and listened to the story of how the tingling and weakness in his legs returned a week after he got home. It got progressively worse until Norman was close to complete paralysis of both legs.

"We need to see your wife and get her version of your illness." McElroy told Norman. He wanted to take a careful history of the home and surroundings. What toxins were in the home? Was the wife also having nerve problems?

A few days later, Norman's wife and mother-in-law came for a visit. Norman had insisted they bring Buddy, his pet Labrador Retriever. They actually brought the dog right up into the ward.

When Dr. McElroy saw the dog, he couldn't believe his eyes: Buddy had no use of his hind legs. The black lab had been fitted with a board on little wheels taped under his belly to support his hind quarters as he walked with his front legs,. All the patients in the ward gathered around to see this dog, who looked like a circus act dragging his little cart on wheels.

McElroy called Barnett into his office to tell him about the partially paralyzed dog. "We've got a man who almost gets well in the hospital, goes home, gets paralyzed again and now brings in a half-paralyzed dog," McElroy said. "There are very few things that can paralyze a man and his dog. Poisons lead the list, and arsenic tops the poisons list." Barnett agreed.

McElroy immediately ordered tests for measuring all poisons in Norman's blood and urine. The test is called "a heavy metal screen." That afternoon, the hospital's maintenance crew showed up with what looked like a big metal fireplace screen and placed it at the foot of Norman's bed. When Dr. McElroy came to do rounds that evening, the first thing he saw was the contraption at the end of Norman's bed. He burst out laughing and couldn't stop. Finally regaining a little composure, he called maintenance. "Well," the man on the phone said, "we don't know what they want it for. Nurse told me to get a heavy metal screen, so that's what we done." McElroy couldn't wait to tell Barnett.

The real heavy metal screening tests on Norman's blood and urine came back. McElroy's suspicion was confirmed: There were very high levels of arsenic.

He shared the results with the patient. This time, Norman wasn't making jokes.

"This weren't no accident, Doc," he said. "Got to be that bitch and her mother who done this. Spiked my food, they did. Hell, I *know* it. Then me feeding my food scraps to poor ol' Buddy got him poisoned, too. They ain't gonna get away with it. They ain't."

Norman was discharged from the hospital and recovered completely. He divorced his wife, who was convicted of attempted murder. She and her mother both went to prison for the crime.

Dr. Barnett told the interns there was a valuable lesson here: "When a man and his dog get sick at the same time, you better think of poisoning."

In this case, both man and dog survived. Buddy also recovered and regained the use of his legs. No longer needing his little makeshift wheeled cart, it remained parked outside the double-wide where Norman lived alone.

Case shared by:

Paul Barnett, M.D.
Associate Clinical Professor of Medicine
Department of Medicine
Vanderbilt University School of Medicine".

Chapter Twenty Three

Remembrance of Things Past
— Marcel Proust*

Dr. Curt Tribble was on call as a senior surgical resident when four adult patients were admitted to the University Burn Unit. He and three other residents were assigned to the patients, each resident caring for one patient. It would be the beginning of two months of nearly constant bedside care for Tribble, who was assigned to the sickest patient. The woman suffered burns over 50 percent of her body.

The first few days of caring for a severe burn are touch and go. The management of fluid replacement demands hourly calculations of the amount and type of intravenous fluid needed. The loss of fluids from the burned areas can be huge, and the need for replacement is critical.

Once the critical early phases pass, then come the needs for surgical wound care followed by skin grafting that goes on for weeks and sometimes months.

Another severe and sometimes fatal problem comes from the extent and nature of the infections that invade the raw area of the burns. The University Burn Unit was well equipped with precise and quantitative measurements of the types of infectious agents in the burned areas. This lab could also determine the exact need for the type and amount of antibiotics to match the infecting agents.

Dr. Tribble's patient became infected with several bacteria, all treated with antibiotics. She also developed an infection with a fungus that led to generalized sepsis, high fevers and early clinical shock. Fungal infections are not treatable with ordinary antibiotics. They require a special drug called amphotericin. This drug must be given in large daily intravenous boluses. It's well known for its toxicity and side effects; at best, it is a tricky drug to administer — so much so that its nickname among surgical residents is "ampho-terrible," an apt name in the case of Tribble's patient.

Each time the calculated dose of amphotericin was given, the patient went into deeper shock with blood pressures falling to very low levels. The infectious disease specialists insisted that the full dose was necessary if the fungus was to be killed. Despite suppressive drugs like Tylenol, Benadryl and cortico- steroids, the drops in blood pressure recurred with each administration of the amphotericin. It appeared she could either die from the fungus or die from the drug or die from both. Something had to be done or the young woman would die in fungal septic shock. She was near terminal.

In the midst of this crisis, Tribble remembered his senior days at Vanderbilt Medical School and being on call every other night in the hospital. One of his favorite spots during down time was the conference room of the department of medicine, located just outside the 24-bed medical inpatient unit. In that room was a filing cabinet that held "blurbs" written by medical residents. As part of their training, each resident was required to write a blurb on a particular subject. Collectively, they were a treasure of clinical information, and Tribble had free access to the short, but informative, jewels during his nights on call. He often spent time reading them and copying many on the nearby copy machine.

Now, somewhere in some remote part of his brain, he recalled reading one of those blurbs about correcting penicillin allergy. He had carefully filed the copies he made those many years ago and still kept them along with hundreds of reprints. Google had nothing on Curt Tribble.

He raced to his on-call room and found the blurb on penicillin allergy. There it was: the details of how to desensitize a patient to penicillin allergy so that penicillin could be used safely. The protocol called for beginning with minute doses of penicillin and progressively increasing the dose, while giving it continuously until the full dose could be tolerated without an allergic reaction.

The big unanswered question was whether or not this method could be used to desensitize the burned patient to the toxic effects of amphotericin. Could a method to deal with an allergic reaction be applied to dealing with a toxic effect of a drug? At first, the attending physicians thought the idea was too far out. But with the young woman near death, they all agreed to try giving the medication continuously, while gradually increasing the dose of amphotericin, just as one would gradually increase the dose of penicillin. This was new clinical ground.

Within a few days, the dose of amphotericin had been increased to the full daily dose, given as a continuous infusion, with no reaction. In a few more days, the steroids and other drugs were stopped. The fever went away and the fungal infection was cured. Although severely scarred from the burns, the young woman survived and was discharged after several months.

As this novel treatment proceeded successfully, Tribble recalled from his youth a memorable admonition from his father, a thoracic surgeon who had often told him stories of his cases. His father's advice, which accompanied most stories, was, "In medicine everything you learn, every story you hear, may be lifesaving. Keep that in mind. This is a very different kind of memory from the tacit lessons of your current education. The lessons of algebra and French can be forgotten with little consequence. Not so with medical knowledge."

Tribble wondered if there is some special part of the brain to store essential clinical information and some indelible neurological recording device to keep it accessible to recall. If so, the recollection of this blurb about desensitization, filed away years earlier and not thought of in the interim, certainly reinforced his father's wisdom from long ago.

Case shared by:

Curt Tribble, MD
Professor of Surgery
Chief, Division of Cardiothoracic Surgery
Vice Chair, Department of Surgery
Medical Director of Transplantation
University of Mississippi

Chapter Twenty Four

Sometimes the cause for a disease can only be heard.*

Janet Sanderford, a mother of three grown sons, was transferred to the University Hospital for increasing shortness of breath. The transferring diagnosis was "suspected mitral valve rupture and pulmonary embolus (blood clots to the lungs)."

Mrs. Sanderford, 58, was accompanied by her husband Jimmy Sanderford, a cattle farmer in southern Indiana. He told the medical resident, "She ain't been no good since that operation."

The operation he was referring to was for a ruptured disc in the spine of her low back. She had undergone the surgery at the local hospital in Indiana about a week before and afterwards had developed swelling in both legs, which was diagnosed as deep vein thrombosis (i.e. clotting of the blood in her leg veins). Deep vein clotting is common after surgery, especially in patients who are obese like Mrs. Sanderford.

Her doctors put her on anticoagulation or blood thinners to prevent further clotting in the veins and to facilitate breakdown of the existing clots.

After a few post-operative days in the local hospital, she had developed increasing severe shortness of breath. It worsened at night, requiring her to sleep upright on pillows. Given her diagnosis of deep vein thrombosis and the possibility of a clot breaking off and going to her lungs, she was transferred to the University Hospital. Just prior to transfer, her surgeon also heard a loud murmur sound from her heart, suggesting the rupture of one of her heart valves. The murmur was not heard during her physical exam before surgery.

On admission to University Hospital, the workup by the medical resident revealed the patient to be short of breath and sitting upright in the bed, preferring to sit on the edge of the bed letting her feet hang freely. Blood pressure was 140/60 and her pulse rate was 92 per minute. She was breathing 24 breaths a minute and appeared frightened and acutely ill. Temperature was normal.

Both legs were swollen to the knees with a large amount of edema (fluid in the tissues). The lungs were moist to listening. There was a loud murmur over the left side of the heart, suggesting mitral valve leakage. The working diagnosis was Congestive Heart Failure due to mitral valve rupture.

The attending physician agreed with the resident and immediately moved Mrs. Sanderford to the cardiac catheterization lab. Both left and right sides of her heart were catheterized. Surprisingly all heart valves were functioning normally with no sign of rupture or leakage. The measured cardiac output of blood was very high at 8.0 liters per minute. Normal is around 3.5 liters per minute.

The attending physician and medical resident were completely mystified to find such a high cardiac output in the face of congestive heart failure. In other words, the heart was failing to pump adequate blood to the body even though it was pumping huge quantities of blood. Something in the body was putting a demand on the heart for more blood than it could pump, i.e. "high output congestive heart failure."

The attending physician called for a cardiac consultation from Dr. Rand Frederiksen. Dr. Frederiksen listened to the story and sequence of events following back surgery. He listened to Mrs. Sanderford's heart and heard the loud murmur. He then noted, as he suspected, that the murmur became louder and louder the lower in the abdomen he moved his stethoscope. The murmur, now a loud swishing sound, was loudest over the right groin, far away from the heart.

Frederiksen turned to the medical resident, "There it is. The arterio-venous or AV fistula is causing the high output failure."

Arteriograms of the aorta and leg vessels showed a connection (fistula) between the right iliac artery and the right iliac vein (vessels moving blood in and out of the right leg). Surgery later that day closed the connection. Mrs. Sanderford recovered completely over the next 48 hours, with no more swelling of her legs or shortness of breath. There were no murmurs heard anywhere in her body.

There are only a few causes for high output heart failure: hyperthyroidism (high thyroid hormone levels), anemia, beri beri from malnutrition and Vitamin B1 deficiency, psoriasis, Paget's disease of Bone, certain forms of liver or kidney disease and arteriovenous fistulas.

The right iliac AV fistula in Mrs. Sanderford's case came from an accidental penetration by the surgeon with a sharp instrument through the disc space from her back into that artery and into the iliac vein, creating a connection. This complication occurs rarely in spine surgery, but it is well known and easily corrected. The surgeon erroneously thought the leg swelling was due to deep vein clotting with later blood clots moving into the lungs, causing the shortness of breath.

The combination of knowing about the particular vascular complication of spine surgery combined with careful listening with the stethoscope lead to the solution of this mystery.

This case was shared by :

Rand T. Frederiksen, M. D.
Clinical Assistant Professor of Medicine (Retired)
Vanderbilt University School of Medicine

Chapter Twenty Five

Labels That Stick *

Josephine Rudolph was referred to Dr. Sidney Warrier with a diagnosis of hypoglycemia, which means recurring low blood sugar. Dr. Warrier was a well known and respected endocrinologist.

There are some diagnoses that most physicians dread to hear, among them hypoglycemia, fibromyalgia and chronic fatigue syndrome. Hypoglycemia leads the list, and Mrs. Rudolph's case is a good example why.

Dr. Warrier had developed his own detective method for dealing with patients who carried a diagnosis of hypoglycemia. The year was 1974. He insisted that Mrs. Rudolph be admitted to the hospital where he could closely observe her over several days. Hospital admissions were easy to obtain in those days; it is too bad that managed care regulations no longer permit such periods of direct observation.

Warrier's plan was quite simple: Every time Mrs. Rudolph had one of her "hypoglycemia" symptoms, she was to call the nurse and have blood drawn for a blood sugar measurement. She was also to record in a bedside diary an exact description of her symptoms and the time of day. This plan would allow direct correlation of Mrs. Rudolph's symptoms with the level of her blood sugar.

When Mrs. Rudolph arrived in her hospital room, she was accompanied by her husband, Frederick Rudolph. Mr. Rudolph carried a large Styrofoam ice chest under each arm, returning with a

93

total of five such chests. After Mrs. Rudolph gave him specific instructions where to place the chests along the wall of the room, she explained to the nurse.

"You see, dear, I have this dreadful allergy to all domestic meats – pork (especially bacon), chicken and beef. I also cannot eat most fish, particularly if raised in ponds. So what do I have to do? I must bring my own meats. I have most of it here for your chef to cook – rabbit, buffalo, pheasant, and quail. My favorite is elk, but it is difficult to find."

Mr. Rudolph made no effort to make social contact and stood by saying nothing. He quietly left the room.

Over the next five days, Mrs. Rudolph reported her symptoms several times a day. By the fifth day, there were 13 entries and 13 blood sugar measurements, occurring at all times of the day.

Some of the recorded symptoms were dizziness, itching all over, extreme weakness, nausea, rapid heartbeat, lightheadedness, blurred vision and pelvic pain.

Dr. Warrier had waited patiently day by day, seeing Mrs. Rudolph each day, listening carefully to her many symptoms but saying nothing except, "Well, let's wait and see what the blood sugars show." He withheld the blood sugar results until he had all of the numbers. On the fifth day, Dr. Warrier pulled a chair to the side of Mrs. Rudolph's bed and placed the results sheet on his lap.

"Mrs. Rudolph, I am glad to tell you that you do not have hypoglycemia. We have these measurements at the height of your symptoms and all the blood sugars are normal – normal being 80 to120. The lowest you showed was 85. I know you must be relieved to see that you do not have hypoglycemia."

Dr. Warrier tilted back in his chair and smiled faintly, visibly satisfied with his plan and presentation.

Mrs. Rudolph paused for several moments, considering all she had just heard. "Well, Dr.Warrier," she began, "I appreciate your thoroughness. But this morning I woke with this terrible itching and scratching feeling in my throat. What do you suggest I take to relieve it?"

Warrier rose from his chair. "Oh, just get one of those over-the-counter gargles or mouthwashes at the drugstore. Use it several times a day, if you need to."

"I can't do that. All those mouthwashes are full of glucose and that would trigger my hypoglycemia," Mrs. Rudolph shot back, raising her nose in the air like she just won the national chess contest.

Dr. Warrier nodded his head slowly, stunned at this woman's denial of the facts and with the failure of his plan to persuade her. He said calmly, "I'll send a full report to your family doctor. He'll know what to do for you." He then headed to the doctors' lounge to tell his colleagues another hypoglycemia story.

The case of Josephine Rudolph is an extreme, but not uncommon, example of patients who carry a diagnosis of hypoglycemia. True hypoglycemia is a very rare condition usually caused by tumors of the pancreas secreting insulin. (See Chapter 14. An Uncommon Cure for a case report.) However, despite the rarity, the false diagnosis or label of hypoglycemia is very common. Many people with the label are also insistent about having the condition. No amount of reassuring or measuring normal blood sugars will dissuade many of these patients or remove the diagnosis.

Over many years somehow the diagnosis began to be applied widely and erroneously to people who had a myriad of vague symptoms even when the blood sugar levels were not low. The problem with any diagnosis, even when false, is that it is nearly impossible to remove the label. One often hears, "But Doctor, so-and-so told me I have hypoglycemia. He must know something that you don't."

Dr. Michael Balint in the 1950s followed and observed a group of family doctors in Scotland and wrote a book called *The Doctor, The Patient, and His Disease.* Balint made the observation that for patients with chronic and unexplained symptoms any label is liable to be permanent, even when the named disease is not present. Diagnoses are difficult to remove.

So it is with hypoglycemia, as well as fibromyalgia and chronic fatigue syndrome. Patients become very attached to their diagnoses, and no amount of evidence to the contrary fazes them.

Dr. Warrier only thought he had a good plan to either substantiate or remove Mrs. Rudolph's diagnosis of hypoglycemia. Obviously, he didn't understand the permanent power of a label, be it true or false.

Case shared by:

Alan Graber, M.D.
Professor of Medicine (retired)
Department of Medicine
Vanderbilt University School of Medicine

Chapter Twenty Six

Learning to Speak
the Language *

Fred Harris, a second-year surgical resident, had just completed his workup on Lummy Jenkins. It was time to present the case findings to fellow residents and faculty surgeon Dr. Curt Tribble, Professor of Thoracic and Cardiovascular Surgery. The group was making rounds on their patients.

When Harris mentioned the name Lummy Jenkins, Tribble interrupted. "So, Lummy is back again. I'm sorry to hear that. Not much left to repair on him. We have repaired or bypassed everything from his carotids to his aorta to his renal arteries. You name it, and Lummy has had it."

"Mr. Jenkins is not here this time for a vascular or cardiac problem," Dr. Harris said, sounding somewhat excited. "He's got an enlarged breast. I think he has breast cancer." The young doctor was obviously proud of his findings and eager for this complex case.

As the group of residents headed into the room, Tribble asked if Harris had questioned Mr. Jenkins about all the drugs that can cause male breast enlargement. Harris had, and Jenkins denied taking any of the medications he named.

Dr. Tribble paused in the hallway. "You did ask him how often he smoked marijuana, didn't you?" Marijuana is a common cause of male breast enlargement (gynecomastia).

Harris frowned. "Mr. Jenkins is an old man from a hollow back in the mountains," he reasoned. "He doesn't smoke marijuana."

Tribble led the group on into the room. "Hey, Lummy. How you been doing?" Jenkins stood by the bedside, smiled a toothless grin and shook Tribble's hand, obviously glad to see him.

"You got a wood shop at your place, right?" Tribble began his questions.

"Yep."

"You have a machine shop too, right?"

"Yep."

"You make a little shine for your own use, right?"

"Yep, just for myself."

"You have a really good garden too, right?"

"Yes, I do."

"Well, like most of the old folks around here, you grow a little of your own marijuana, just for yourself, right?"

"Yep. How did you know that?"

"Lummy, I have known you a long time and I know where you come from."

The two men laughed together.

In the hallway, Tribble turned to Harris. "I suspect we now know the source of his breast enlargement — not by tests but by a simple, human conversation. I did several things in there with Lummy to get vital information. I let him know I knew his culture and some details of that. I also chose the first questions to make him comfortable and get positive answers. That let him know it was OK to say "yes." Then I phrased the last question so he could answer honestly without worrying. I entered the world of Lummy Jenkins, and he let me into it.

"Of course we will get an estrogen level just to be sure he does not have an estrogen secreting tumor somewhere," Dr. Tribble continued. "Assuming those tests are negative, we can expect the breast to shrink on its own if he stops or reduces smoking marijuana. But at his age, I doubt if Lummy will do either. That's up to him."

Editor's Note:

Dr. Tribble used several techniques to gain rapport. Entering the world of the patient is essential. Sometimes shifting voice tones to match the patient will help. When attempting to get sensitive or delicate information, it is necessary to give permission for an admission of a noxious habit. For example, when attempting to get an accurate laxative history in patients with low blood potassium levels and suspected laxative abuse, one might frame the question this way:

"Mr./Ms. (name), we all use laxatives some time. I have patients who take only one bottle of milk of magnesia a day and I have some who take up to five bottles a day. How much do you take?"

By leading up to the mention of marijuana, Tribble was permitting "yes" answers to private information. The careful questioning saved Lummy from an unnecessary mastectomy.

*Case shared by:

Curt Tribble, MD
Professor of Surgery
Chief, Division of Cardiothoracic Surgery
Vice Chair, Department of Surgery
Medical Director of Transplantation
University of Mississippi

Chapter Twenty Seven

Sometimes the Answer to a Single Question Solves the Mystery *

Gilford Matthe was a drug rep for a national pharmaceutical company. He and his wife lived in Gainesville, Florida. He called on gynecologists mostly, introducing new drug products for women and promoting the company's line of drugs and hormones. He periodically visited Dr. Madeline Simmons, a gynecologist with a large referral practice. Dr. Simmons was a professor of gynecology at the regional medical center and medical school. Her specialty included infertility.

On one of his visits, Gilford asked if Dr. Simmons would see him and his wife for a fertility workup. They had been married for several years and had been unable to get pregnant. They had wanted a child since they first married, but hadn't had a fertility workup to find out why they had not yet conceived.

When his wife Janice came in for the appointment, Dr. Simmons explained the fertility workup and asked if there were any questions. Janice shook her head "no," so the workup began. After an exhaustive set of questions about her menstrual history and general medical history, Dr. Simmons began a complete physical and pelvic exam. Both were normal. Samples of the cervical mucous and lining of the uterus were sent for microscopic evaluation. These, too, were normal.

The next phase of the workup required a variety of hormone measurements in Janice's blood. Ovarian function is controlled by the pituitary gland in the brain, so Dr. Simmons measured these controlling hormones, as well as thyroid hormone levels. All showed normal levels. The cause for infertility was still missing.

The next phase required a detailed study of the anatomy of the uterus and the fallopian tubes that led to the ovaries. These tubes carry the mother's eggs down from the ovaries into the body of the uterus for union with the male sperm. A dye is injected into the uterus for x-ray examination to see if the dye is transmitted into the fallopian tubes. A blocked fallopian tube is one common cause for failure to conceive; the egg cannot get to the body of the uterus. This particular test must be done either late or very early in the menstrual cycle when there is little chance of interfering with a pregnancy. The test has a long name: hysterosalpingogram. Janice's test was normal, ruling out tubal blockage as the cause of infertility.

The final evaluation included additional uterine tissue sampling and daily temperatures to see if ovulation was occurring. Both of these were also normal. The results of the complete workup revealed Janice Matthe to be a potentially fertile woman.

Dr. Simmons then turned her attention to Gilford Matthe. His detailed medical history revealed no serious illnesses and no surgery. There had been no injuries to his testicles, and he had never had mumps that might have infected his testicles. His physical exam profiled a normal adult male with no signs of testosterone (male hormone) deficiency. A sperm count revealed healthy and normally mobile sperm.

At this point, Dr. Simmons was stumped. She called the couple in to lay out her plans for the next, most complicated phase of a fertility program that involved timed copulation tied to daily temperature measurements. As she began the lengthy description, a question popped into her head.

"How often do you have sexual intercourse?" she asked.

"Oh, we haven't had sex in several years," Gilford answered. Janice said nothing.

The answer floored Dr. Simmons — and still does.

After several awkward moments waiting some further comment from either Gilford or Janice, Dr. Simmons finally said, "Well, then, I think we have our answer to your infertility." With that, the couple rose and walked out of the exam room. She never saw them again.

Dr. Simmons sat puzzling over the entire encounter and the unnecessary fertility workup. She asked herself why a well-informed man would seek an expensive and lengthy fertility workup in the face of a long period of sexual abstinence. She raised a multitude of unanswered questions that might explain the bizarre behavior: Was Janice frigid and Gilford thought this might lead Dr. Simmons to discover and address the problem? Was Gilford impotent and embarrassed to discuss it? Why didn't the wife raise any question? Could there be some sexual deviancy that Gilford wanted the doctor to unearth and resolve?

But the most important question was raised by Dr. Simmons's reflection: "Why didn't I think to ask them how often they had intercourse before the workup?"

We will never know the true answer about their motives. One thing is certain in this case, however: The answer to a single question can solve a lot of mysteries. Dr. Simmons says her first question in any infertility workup, now embedded in her brain, is "When and how often do you have intercourse?" Every time she asks the question, she remembers the Matthes and still wonders what they were thinking.

Case shared by:

Betty Ruth Speir, M.D.
Adjunct Professor of Obstetrics and Gynecology
Professor Emerita of General Surgery
University of South Alabama College of Medicine

Chapter Twenty Eight

*Strange Intuition ***

Late one day in October, Wilbur Cleaves called Dr. Paul Barnett's office and insisted on speaking to the doctor. Wilbur had been a patient of Barnett's for many years and had a close relationship with him. Except for mild, treated high blood pressure, Cleaves was in good health. The phone call was about his wife, Caroline, who just turned 47.

Caroline had just been diagnosed with a malignant lymphoma by her home doctor in Kentucky. Wilbur wanted her to see Dr. Barnett. Barnett told him she really should be under the care of an oncologist to guide her treatment and offered to make a phone call on her behalf, but Wilbur declined.

"Don't ask me how I know," Wilbur told the doctor. "I just know Caroline does not have any lymphoma. I somehow know it. Caroline just doesn't look like she has any cancer."

The two men talked a while longer, and Wilbur remained steadfast. Barnett figured this insistence there was no cancer was simply denial by an upset husband, which is not uncommon. Barnett decided to see Caroline, knowing he would have her seen by an oncologist at the same time.

When Caroline arrived to see Dr. Barnett, Barnett had the resident do the initial medical workup. He found she had weight loss of 10 pounds, low-grade fever and large lymph nodes in her neck. The chest x-ray also showed enlarged nodes behind her sternum.

All blood chemistries and blood counts were normal. The diagnosis seemed firmly established, since a biopsy of a node had showed changes of a lymphoma. The only notable factor in her past history was a history of grand mal epileptic seizures beginning more than 10 years ago. Caroline had been taking Dilantin (phenytoin) daily with good control of the seizures.

Dr. Claude Wills, the medical resident, called Barnett to report his examination and history. "Looks like she's got a lymphoma to me. However, I just read a report about pseudolymphomas being caused by Dilantin. Guess we ought to check that out." (See Chapter Notes.)

Barnett thanked the resident and could not wait to read the reported case of pseudolymphoma caused by Dilantin. It was the first he had heard of the syndrome. As so often happens, interns and residents are reading the medical literature voraciously. Often they read of new diseases and treatments before the faculty.

Given Wilbur's refusal to accept a diagnosis of lymphoma in his wife, Barnett suggested stopping the Dilantin first before beginning any chemotherapy. He would see what would happen to the lymph nodes. By the end of six months, all nodes returned to normal size, the fever went away and Caroline regained her weight. Young Dr. Wills had come across the key information. The diagnosis was established as "phenytoin-induced pseudolymphoma."

Barnett's review of the literature found two different syndromes of Dilantin associated lymph node enlargement. The first syndrome, the rarest, occurs shortly after beginning Dilantin treatment. It is now called the "anticonvulsant hypersensitivity syndrome" and is associated with fever, rash, enlarged nodes and hepatitis. It usually begins within eight weeks of beginning Dilantin treatment.

The second syndrome, as in this case with Caroline Cleaves, is called "phenytoin-induced pseudolymphoma." It is slow to develop, coming even years after being on Dilantin. Both syndromes vanish on stopping the drug.

It is clear that the resident from his readings led Dr. Barnett to the correct diagnosis. What remains a mystery is how the husband knew to reject the diagnosis of a malignant lymphoma.

One can only wonder what tragic course would have occurred had chemotherapy been initiated.

Case shared by:

Paul Barnett, M.D.
Associate Clinical Professor of Medicine
Department of Medicine
Vanderbilt University School of Medicine".

Chapter Twenty Nine

"Extratebreastrial" Communication *

Tiffany Snopes, a 31-year-old woman, was first seen in the Surgery Clinic of University Hospital complaining of problems with her breast implants.

Dr. J. Willis Malone, a plastic surgeon, asked Ms. Snopes to describe the problem.

She rambled on for the better part of 10 minutes about her insomnia and unwanted weight loss, then began describing — in great and unnecessary detail — her long trip to Singapore three years ago where she had the implants inserted. Her tale went on for at least 15 more minutes, chock full of digressions and trivia that no one, especially this busy doctor, wanted to hear.

Dr. Malone interrupted politely, "Please, Ms. Snopes, could you tell me what the problem is?"

She paused and blinked for a moment, as if trying to understand the question.

"Well," she finally said with some indignation, "I haven't had one moment's peace since they put those things in me. I cannot sleep. I cannot think. It is incessant. I want them removed _now_."

"Can you *describe* the problem?" he asked. "Is it pain? Do they hurt you? Are they too small or too large? I need more information before I can help you." Malone was getting frustrated.

"All night long they go on," she continued, hardly taking a breath. "It's those Martians. My breast implants are audio devices for the Martians. Didn't I tell you that? They talk to each other all the time. Sometimes they yell and wake me up. I can't stand this anymore. I want these implants out so I can get some peace and quiet!"

Malone stood there dumbfounded. At first he thought someone had put her up to this as a joke. It was beyond outrageous. But he could clearly see she was very serious and very upset. He had never encountered anything like it. The woman was obviously delusional and paranoid.

The more he listened and questioned her, the more he was convinced these delusions and paranoia were highly selective and limited. She was not worried about a whole host of things, as is often the case. Her paranoia was focused exclusively on aliens using her breast implants as communication devices.

Malone called in Dr. Sidney Mayhand for psychiatric consultation. After lengthy interviews with Ms. Snopes, Mayhand was convinced there could be no psychological progress until the implants were removed. He told Dr. Malone he had seen people with very limited delusions like this before, but none had centered on breast implants.

"She is refusing any kind of psychiatric treatment or drugs until the implants are removed," Mayhand said. "I know it is heterodoxy, but I suggest you comply with her request and remove the implants."

"Are you nuts?" Malone replied. "Me? Remove implants from a psychotic woman? I can imagine the jury now. There's no telling what a lawyer would try to get out of me for that. They would have a field day!"

Dr. Mayhand tried once again to convince Ms. Snopes that medications would stop her delusions, but she adamantly refused to take them. She didn't need them, she said. All efforts to convince her otherwise fell on deaf ears.

Running out of options, Mayhand and Malone asked to meet with the hospital's ethics committee and attorneys to discuss the situation. After careful consideration, all parties supported a plan to remove the implants as the only treatment that might give the patient relief, noting in the record that her general health was deteriorating from the insomnia and weight loss. Legal consent forms were drawn up and signed by witnesses, the patient herself and an uncle, who was her only living relative.

Dr. Malone, still reluctant, scheduled surgery. In her terms, she demanded "American breast implants and get rid of these Singapore things."

After the procedure, Ms. Snopes woke from the anesthesia. Immediately, she seemed a different person, smiling and happy. When Dr. Malone made his first post -op visit, she was sitting on the edge of her bed.

"Oh, thank goodness!" she exclaimed when she saw him. "It's the first time in over two years those voices have shut up. Thank you, thank you so much."

Malone told her he was glad she had relief and took the opportunity of her good humor to remind her of the promise she made to continue to see Dr. Mayhand for psychiatric treatment. "Now don't go back on your word," he said.

"But Dr. Malone," she said, still smiling, "you cured me. I don't need any more treatment. You fixed it!"

Ms. Snopes went home on the third post-op day, staying longer than usual to allow for some follow-up. She refused to see Dr. Mayhand. She was never seen again. No one ever knew how long her delusions or paranoia remained in remission. All they knew for sure was that she remained free of the alien voices for those three happy days.

This case was shared by a colleague who wishes to remain anonymous.

Chapter Thirty

The Honeymoon

By Sidney R. Block, M.D.

"I can't breathe", is what Martha actually said, but in the middle of Stage IV sleep, what I heard (or thought I heard) was, "I can't sleep." As I slowly stumbled up the cognitive staircase to awareness but not yet at the step of comprehension, she repeated, "I can't breathe", and, now in Stage I, I dreamed she was saying once again, "I can't sleep." "So," I warned myself in my preawakened stupor, "this is what marriage is all about: she can't sleep and I need to be told about it."

It was the second night of our marriage, the first having been spent in the Honeymoon Suite of the Plaza in New York City, and even that notwithstanding we had managed a reasonably restful number of hours of sleep before arising and leaving the next morning for a villa on the coast of Bermuda which offered wonderful views, great privacy and a breakfast served on our patio overlooking the Atlantic Ocean.

"I can't breathe", Martha now strained to implore with greater urgency, and now fully awake, I also could discern her anxiety and evident respiratory distress. Sans stethoscope, I had to listen to her chest, an exercise which during a honeymoon should have been a pleasurable effort. Hearing only a mild tachycardia and no adventitious sounds and everything else between her heart and my ear seeming to be in perfect order (in retrospect I should have sat her up first and put my ear to the back of her chest—-but, again, it was our honeymoon, and though accordingly I have ever since forgiven myself, she has not), I helped her sit up and lean forward which seemed to help. I tried to be of further assistance by propping her up even more with the available pillows. She didn't worsen but she also didn't improve much, and we remained awake and concerned until daybreak.

After getting out of bed and sitting on the patio waiting for breakfast to arrive, there was evident improvement in her respirations and we relaxed a bit. The maid arrived with a large tray full of fresh coffee, pastries, eggs and fruit, and after setting our table, looked at us and noted that though we looked tired (as well we should have been on the second night of our marriage), we did not look as happy as she would have expected.

The maid inquired about how we had spent the night.

Martha replied, "Not well; I had trouble breathing."

"Oh, do you have any allergies?"

"Only to feathers."

"Well then, just let me take those down pillows and replace them for you," and she left to do just that.

My wife gave me a look, a look that included a wry smile (a look that I have come to know much better over the last 43 years). "A lot of good it did me, did it, marrying a doctor!"

Story told by:

Sidney R. Block, M.D.
Northport, Maine

Chapter Thirty One

A Case of Overkill *

May Cusins was a 78 year old woman admitted for pneumonia. This was her third admission for pneumonia in the past year.

Dr. Allen Kaiser, an infectious disease consultant, had been asked to see Mrs. Cusins to see if he could uncover any cause for her repeated bouts with pneumonia. Lung scans and a bronchoscopy on a previous admission had been unrevealing.

Dr. Kaiser, with his team of a medical resident, an intern, and three junior medical students entered the room. He introduced the team to Mrs. Cusins.

"Mrs. Cusins, your doctor asked me to see you about your pneumonia. We need to ask you some questions. "

"Well go right ahead." Mrs. Cusins had no teeth so she gummed her mouth up and down as she talked.

"Do you live in town?" Kaiser asked.

"Oh no. I live way up in the country. Out from Jamestown. Live in a trailer with Hunt. He's my husband. Been married 61 years."

"I see. I need to go down a list of things. Any dust around your place?"

"Nope."

"Any blackbird roosts nearby?"

"Nope. Aint' no trees."

"Use any insecticides?" Kaiser was moving from one inhalant to another.

Mrs. Cusins looked puzzled, hesitated, then said, "Don't think so."

"Are you sure?" Kaiser pressed on, not certain she understood the word. With no response, he asked, "Got in any insects in your trailer?"

"Aint no insects but it's full of roaches. Some of 'em an inch long." she responded.

"What do you do about the roaches?"

About that time, Mr. Cusins came into the room. Mrs. Cusins said, "Hunt, tell 'em about the roaches."

"Hell every time she gets out the cans of 'Real Kill', I have to run out the trailer. She don't use just one can. She uses 2 cans."

Kaiser turned to his team and smiled. "Real Kill, like all insecticide sprays contains pyrithrene or a derivative molecule. It is neurotoxic to all insects. Also toxic to the lungs of humans if they are allergic or sensitive to it."

Hunt Cusins turned to his wife. "I told you one can was enough. I knowed those 2 cans was too much."

Kaiser said, "Sooner or later if you keep asking, you will get the answer. Patients like Mrs. Cusins often know the answer but we have to teach each other our names for things. Takes a bit of patience. Everything has a cause."

Case shared b:

Allen Kaiser, M.D.
Chief of Staff
Vanderbilt Health System
Professor of Medicine, Vanderbilt University

Chapter Thirty Two

*Some Mysteries Remain Mysteries**

Alfred Lee Henderson always came to clinic with his wife. Both were over dressed and looked a bit out of place in the clinic waiting room.

Alfred Lee wore two tone black and white wing tipped shoes – Spectator shoes. His suit was black with cream pin stripes, as was his matching vest. He tied his tie in a large Winsor knot. He looked like a movie version of a Wall Street Banker.

His wife, Sarah Elizabeth, was beautiful with long brunette hair swept to one side of her head. She was nearly six feet tall. Whenever the two walked into the clinic waiting room they drew the full attention of waiting patients. An audible hum rippled across the group.

Dr. Allen Kaiser, an infectious disease specialist, was seeing Alfred Lee Henderson for the first time. Both Henderson and his wife were waiting in the small exam room when Kaiser entered. Henderson had been referred to Dr. Kaiser by a primary care provider who had been treating Mr. Henderson for several months for recurring abscesses on his arm. He now required a PICC line (Peripherally Inserted Central Catheter) for IV antibiotics. New abscesses continued to appear and the frustrated primary care provider referred him to Dr. Kaiser for advice.

There were many reports in Henderson's medical record of the cultures of the abscess pus. The large number and variety of types of different microorganisms (bacteria) was something Kaiser had not seen before. Usually abscesses grow out a single organism such as staphylococcus. In Henderson's case, there were half dozen different bacteria. Some were not classifiable, simply labeled "gram positive rod, not classifiable".

All of the extensive laboratory test results were normal. Efforts to examine the immune system, including a HIV test were normal.

Dr. Kaiser had difficulty drawing either Henderson or his wife into any sort of dialogue. They either answered with one syllable or they nodded their heads in yes or no responses. He did glean with some difficulty that Henderson worked in a bank in a small town in Alabama. No, he was not an officer in the bank. Yes, he was a clerk and book keeper in the bank. (Kaiser was a bit surprised, expecting Henderson to be at least an officer in the bank.)

Kaiser got nowhere is searching for unusual contacts with plants or wild animals as a source of infecting agents. Henderson said his daily activities were unchanged from the time before the abscesses began.

After half an hour, Kaiser, drawing a blank, ended the interview. His physical examination found a dozen or more abscesses from the shoulder to the top of the hand. They were only on the left arm and hand. He did note that Henderson was right handed. The rest of the physical examination was normal.

Puzzled by his failure to make rapport with the couple, Kaiser reviewed the social worker notes. There he found that the couple, although still married, no longer lived together. No reason was given for living apart. Both always attended the clinic together. The social worker also had difficulty drawing the couple into conversation.

Henderson returned to clinic in one week. Dr. Kaiser had formulated his plan. He engaged the head nurse to come with him into the exam room as a witness. Fearing some anger and even possible retribution for what he was about to say, he placed a voice recorder in his coat pocket and turned it on.

Kaiser sat at the desk in the small exam room and faced the couple sitting off to his right. He introduced the nurse.

Then, in a most serious monotone, Kaiser began his talk. "I have thought long and hard about your problems with the abscesses on your left arm. I must be completely honest with you. It will be no help at all if we continue this false guise of pretending you have some obscure disease. I am certain of one thing. I am certain that you are injecting or rubbing something into your left arm to cause the abscesses. You are right handed. The abscesses are only on the left arm. From the mixture of bacteria, you are either rubbing saliva or dirt or feces into the left arm."

Kaiser, the nurse witness, and both Henderson's sat in silence for several minutes. Kaiser, in telling this case story, said his heart was pounding, not knowing what to expect. After a few more minutes, both Henderson's rose and walked out of the exam room, saying nothing... nothing.

Dr. Kaiser never saw the Henderson's again. He did hear months later from their local family doctor that the abscesses had cleared from Henderson's arm.

There is an old dictum about self induced injuries or infections. It says, "The doctor who makes the diagnosis of self infliction will never be the doctor who treats it." That is so true. Whenever the relationship drops to that level of deception and lack of trust, there can be no healing doctor-patient relationship.

Case shared by:

Allen Kaiser, M.D.
Chief of Staff
Vanderbilt Health System
Professor of Medicine, Vanderbilt University

Chapter Thirty Three

A Case of the Blues *

Jake Deacon rode motorcycles with his Harley Club every weekend. Even though he spent his weekdays as a truck driver, to him there was nothing like the feeling of traveling those same open roads on his motorcycle. He loved to ride.

In the late spring of 1984, Deacon was cruising a Tennessee back road between Memphis and Jackson when his motorcycle spun out on a curve. His body slid more than 30 yards across the gritty asphalt. His leathers offered little protection.

The skin over the right side of his body was severely abraded. The femur and tibia of his right leg were badly fractured, exposing the bones of his thigh and lower leg.

He was airlifted to the University Hospital in Memphis and admitted to the Intensive Care Unit.

After multiple orthopedic procedures, skin grafts and a three-month stay in a rehab unit, Deacon was finally discharged to his home near Nashville. It had been a long and painful process, but his injuries were healing. He was grateful to be alive and looked forward to getting back to his life.

Back home, Deacon's health didn't continue to improve as he hoped. He remained in constant pain — not just where he was injured, but throughout his body. He spiraled into depression and suffered from a profound lack of energy.

Driving a truck was no longer possible, so he quit and applied to Social Security for disability. This led to an extensive psychiatric evaluation, which labeled him as "malingering and seeking money for his alleged but unproven disability." His claim was denied.

Deacon began seeing different doctors, hoping someone could diagnose and cure what he knew to be a very real physical debility. Among the many who saw him, there were diverse opinions about the cause for his continued troubles. Some believed he had severe depression, but trials on antidepressants failed to give any relief. Others believed he had chronic fatigue syndrome, while still others thought he had some obscure malignancy yet to surface. This latter diagnosis stemmed from the fact that lymph nodes in his neck and under his arm were tender. But a biopsy showed no abnormality of the nodes.

In fact, all tests revealed normal values. There was no evidence for liver, heart, kidney, gastrointestinal or neurological diseases. Repeated measurements also remained normal.

Deacon continued to describe himself as "just feeling sick." He said he woke in the morning feeling somewhat better than when he went to bed. As the day wore on, he felt sicker and sicker. He suspected he often had a low-grade fever, but an elevated temperature was never documented. He also reported having an itchy rash from time to time, but no doctor ever saw it.

His major complaint was aching in all his major joints. Deacon consulted a rheumatologist who ordered tests for known joint or soft tissue diseases. All were normal. A biopsy of his calf muscle revealed no inflammation of his small blood vessels, ruling out a number of types of vasculitis.

It had now been two years since Deacon's motorcycle accident. He remained unemployed, undiagnosed and chronically ill.

He was referred to see Dr. Paul Barnett, a general internist known for his diagnostic abilities in patients with obscure and undefined symptoms. Dr. Barnett repeated most of the tests Deacon had been given, and results were still normal. Over the course of several weeks, the doctor explored the habits and psychological aspects of Deacon's life and found no stressors to account for the chronic complaints. Deacon had a solid marriage and two healthy children. Although he was unemployed, his wife made enough money to support the family. Again, a dead end for any explanation of Deacon's complaints.

One day, Deacon came in to see Barnett and sat directly across the desk from the doctor. Barnett squinted at Deacon. "What's that white streak on your chin?" he asked.

Deacon rubbed his chin, smiled and said, "Oh that's just some blue cheese dressing. I love the stuff. Eat a salad with it almost every day."

Barnett leaned forward in his chair, considering a new possibility. He asked Deacon to tell him, in detail, exactly how much and how often he ate blue cheese. The answer was, literally, "Every day."

"Let's try a long shot," the doctor said. "Hold off the blue cheese and let's see what happens. Don't eat any — not one little bit."

Well, this was by far the weirdest "prescription" Deacon had gotten from all the many doctors he'd seen. But he was willing to try anything to feel better and agreed to stay away from his favorite food.

Deacon came back a week early for his next appointment. He was so excited, he couldn't wait to see Dr. Barnett. "I'm completely well," he blurted out as soon as the good doctor walked in the room. "Wake up normal. Ready to go. No more aching anywhere. Tender lumps in my neck? Gone. Sleep through the night. I'm even applying for my truck driving job. It's a miracle, Doc."

Since his last visit with Deacon, Barnett had done some research to confirm what he suspected when he heard about his patient's blue cheese habit. Sure enough, he found that the smelly, moldy cheese contains either Penicillin roqueforti or Penicillin glaucum. Both molds release a form of penicillin. Dr. Barnett knew that constant penicillin in the bloodstream can produce serum sickness from a chronic immune response. Deacon had a case of serum sickness.

Serum sickness is caused by the immune system responding to something in the blood that it "sees" as abnormal. Immune complexes form and cause inflammation in the joints, lymph nodes and sometimes small blood vessels. Antitoxin sera of various sorts can also cause the reaction. Antibiotics are known causes, penicillin most often listed.

The symptoms can be partially relieved by corticosteroids or non-steroidal anti-inflammatory agents. All symptoms usually go away within a week of stopping the offending drug or agent. The symptoms return if the drug is taken again.

An extensive search of the medical literature fails to find even one other case of serum sickness caused by blue cheese. Most people consume blue cheese intermittently, but Jake Deacon's daily consumption created a sustained blood level of penicillin, thus triggering the immune response and serum sickness. This is believed to be the only case of serum sickness from blue cheese.

"I was cured within a week after I stopped eating blue cheese," Deacon said. "Who ever thought that all this time of being sick would be caused by eating a salad I thought was good for me?"

Case shared by

Paul Barnett, M.D.
Associate Clinical Professor of Medicine
Department of Medicine
Vanderbilt University School of Medicine".

Chapter Thirty Four

Open and Shut Case *

Editor Note: This highly technical case illustrates the extraordinary diagnostic power when knowledge in physiology and technology are combined. The solution to this case required both.

Chronic pain in Lester Littler's fingers and knees was the first sign something wasn't right. The 62-year-old mechanic and farmer also noticed slight swelling and redness at his joints, but he wasn't particularly alarmed.

He happened to mention this to his family doctor, Dr. Moore, who wasn't alarmed either. He thought Littler might have mild rheumatoid or osteoarthritis and prescribed Motrin.

The Motrin provided some relief at first, but over a three-month period the joint pains increased. Littler returned to see his doctor. Now thinking the joint pain might be gout, Dr. Moore tested blood uric acid level. He also tested for rheumatoid arthritis. Both came back normal.

At this visit, Dr. Moore noticed something else: Littler's fingernails appeared unnaturally curved and rounded. It looked like a classic case of "clubbing," which can be caused by a number of diseases, some of them dire. The doctor ordered x-rays for both chest and bones.

The chest x-ray revealed a nodule the size of a golf ball in Littler's left lung. The bone x-rays revealed inflammation and elevation of the covering of the bones, the so-called periosteal layer on the surface of the bones. This condition is called "hypertrophic osteoarthropathy." It is a rare manifestation of lung cancer, as is the clubbing of the fingernails.

Littler underwent surgery in which lung cancer was found and his entire left lung removed. There was no evidence for the cancer spreading.

Immediately after surgery, Littler's knees and hands started to feel normal again. The pain and inflammation he had experienced disappeared completely over about two weeks; his fingernails soon returned to normal.

The clinical story up to this point was relatively simple: Lester Littler had a rare manifestation of lung cancer, the lung cancer was removed and the symptoms of painful joints and clubbing disappeared.

But then things began to get complicated.

Littler recovered nicely from the operation and, after two weeks, was back doing mild chores on the farm. About six weeks after the operation, however, he started feeling short of breath on his daily routine activities. This worsened until walking fast or going up stairs carrying loads made him uncomfortably short of breath.

He went back to Dr. Moore whose exam could find no reason for Littler's distress. Yet he had a respiratory rate well above normal, the normal rate of breathing being 10 to 12 breaths per minute. Littler was breathing 18 times a minute just sitting quietly in the exam room.

The doctor did pulmonary function tests which revealed only the expected loss of lung volume due to the removal of his left lung. But this did not explain his rapid breathing. A CT angiogram of the arteries to the lung showed no evidence for an embolus (clot in the pulmonary artery), and his blood count was normal, ruling out anemia as an explanation for the shortness of breath.

The Moore had no answers, but noted that Littler's oxygen saturation was 88%, whereas normal is 95%. He decided to begin Littler on 2 liters of nasal oxygen at home, to see if his breathing improved.

Over the next several weeks, the shortness of breath worsened. Littler was now breathing over 30 breaths a minute. Unable to get from his bed to the bathroom without unbearable shortness of breath, he went to the local ER on a Sunday afternoon.

The ER physician, lacking any explanation, called Dr. John Newman at Vanderbilt Medical Center for a pulmonary consultation. In the local ER, Littler's oxygen saturation was only 75%. This did not rise even when the nasal oxygen was raised to 10 liters per minute, the maximum deliverable via the nasal catheter. Littler was saying over and over that he would blow his brains out if he did not get relief soon. He was having terrible headaches and mild chest pains on top of the extreme shortness of breath.

Dr. Newman quickly reviewed the other findings. The chest x-ray showed the expected fluid in the left chest where the cancerous lung had been removed. The right lung was normal, with no pneumonia or sign of abnormal arteries or veins.

Newman then suggested the local ER doctor give Littler an oxygen mask which would deliver pure oxygen at a 100% level. When the ER doctor reported back that Littler's saturation was only 78% while breathing 100% pure oxygen, Dr. Newman knew the answer to their puzzle.

Recalling basic respiratory physiology, he knew a low oxygen saturation in the face of breathing 100% oxygen meant only one thing: the presence of an arterio-venous shunt. The low oxygen containing venous blood was going directly into the arteries without passing the oxygen sacs in the lung, a so-called "right to left shunt" of blood. In other words, the blood was getting through the chest without being exposed to oxygen in the lung alveoli and then passing into the body with very low oxygen levels. In effect, the body was barely staying alive on nearly pure venous blood.

Dr. Newman was sure there must be a shunt bypassing the lung, but where was it? Littler was transferred to the Intensive Care Unit at Vanderbilt Medical Center. When he arrived, he was breathing 30 breaths a minute, sitting up straight in bed. He had constant chest pain. An echocardiogram (EKG) at the bedside showed no hole in the heart, and even with injection of saline with small bubbles as tracers, there was no visible shunt. The small bubbles passed directly into the arteries of the lungs as they do normally. No shunt was found by this method.

Now the case really gets complicated. All evidence says there must be a shunt from right to left from veins to arteries somewhere in the chest. Otherwise the 100 percent oxygen would have increased the oxygen level in Littler's blood.

Still convinced there had to be a shunt despite failure to show it with the echocardiogram, Dr. Newman insisted on a full cardiac catheterization – the absolute gold standard for looking for a shunt. At catheterization, as suspected, there it was: an open hole between the two atria of the heart known as the foramen ovale, a vestige from fetal life when the foramen ovale is open. The case is solved. The surgical closure of the foramen ovale will cure the problem.

Here we need a short digression. Before birth, the infant has no need for oxygen from the lungs, because oxygen comes from its mother's blood in the placenta. So the blood from the lungs is bypassed through a hole in baby's heart. That hole is the foramen ovale. At birth, the hole in the heart miraculously closes, and venous blood then flows into the arteries of the baby's lungs where it receives the oxygen breathed in by the infant. Littler's foramen ovale, closed since birth, was forced open from the rotation and twisting of his remaining right lung into the space of the removed left lung. This allowed the venous blood to flow into the arterial side, thus shunting the blood away from the oxygen in the lungs.

But why did the echocardiogram fail to reveal the shunt? The answer: The saline tracer was injected into an arm vein. Blood that traversed the foramen ovale was streaming up from the leg and abdominal veins via the inferior vena cava. Blood from the arm veins passes directly into the artery to the lung failing to reveal the open foramen ovale.

Littler was taken to the OR by the thoracic surgeons and the open foramen ovale was confirmed and sutured closed. The arterial oxygen level returned to normal within a few minutes of the closure.

Knowledge of basic physiology permitted an accurate solution to this case: Breathing pure oxygen raises the oxygen content of blood unless there is an arterio-venous shunt. But the sequence of events were most uncommon, there being only five reported cases of a foramen ovale opening after lung resection.

As for Littler, he returned to his farm and never had another problem with his lung.

Case shared by:

John Newman, M.D.
Elsa S. Hanigan Professor of Pulmonary Medicine
Division of Pulmonary and Critical Care Medicine
Department of Medicine
Vanderbilt University School of Medicine

Chapter Thirty Five

*Itch in a College Student ***

Fred Orville was winding down his last week in college. The last few weeks had been filled with all night parties and "serious drinking," as he liked to say.

For over a month, Fred noticed a rash begin to appear on his legs and arms. Sometimes it looked like hives but then it changed into small raised plaques. The itching became intolerable so he went to the Student Health Center where he was given calomel lotion and some Benadryl to take by mouth. They told him he was allergic to something he had touched.

The drugs gave him no relief and the itching increased. So did the area of the rash. He now had lesions inside his mouth and over his entire body. He had to get some relief. The Student Health nurse got him an appointment with the Dermatology Clinic the next day.

Dr. Michael Jenkins met Fred in his exam room, took one look at the skin lesions and said, "You've got lichen planus. That's for sure. Of course I will biopsy to be certain."

Jenkins did not tell Fred that sometimes the lichen planus lesions can predispose to the development of skin cancer (squamous cell type.)

Fred kept saying, "I've got to get some relief. Can you do something to stop this itching?"

Dr. Jenkins told Fred he would start him on oral cortisone-like steroids and see him in a week with the biopsy report. Jenkins took a small biopsy on Fred's arm.

By the second day of steroids, Fred's itching was much less and he was free of the itch by the fourth day. The biopsy confirmed the diagnosis of lichen planus and showed no evidence for skin cancer.

Dr. Jenkins was glad to hear that the itching had been relieved. He explained to Fred that most cases of lichen planus are "idiopathic", meaning the cause is unknown. He went on to name a long list of substances known to cause the disease. The list included anti-malarial drugs, penicillamine, thiazide diuretics, beta blockers, non-steroidal anti-inflammatory agents, quinidine, angiotensin-converting enzyme inhibitors, or gold containing compounds. The disease also has been linked to hepatitis C viral infections.

"Fred, it's our shared job to see if we can uncover a cause. I want you to keep a daily diary of all you eat or drink and notes about locations or other observations. Let's see if we can find the culprit."

Fred brought his diary with him on his next visit. There was nothing on the list that suggested it as a cause of the skin lesions. Suddenly Fred sat up straight with a new thought. "I think I may have it. I drank a lot of cinnamon schnapps this past year. We called it the "gold drink." Do you suppose it's really got gold in it?"

Dr. Jenkins told Fred to bring in a bottle and they would find out. Later, when several bottles were analyzed there were 8 to 17 metallic flakes per 750 liter bottle. The metallic flakes were 75% gold by weight, with 280 micrograms of gold per deciliter dissolved in the liquid.

Measurements of Fred's blood and urine showed a serum level of gold to be 0.4 mg per liter (normal range 0 to 0.1). His 24 hour urine specimen showed 86 micrograms of gold (normal range 0 to 1.0 microgram). These measurements were made three months after Fred's last drink of gold schnapps. Three months later the blood and urine gold levels were within the normal range.

The skin lesions and itching gradually disappeared as Fred avoided drinking the gold schnapps.

Fred was heard to say, "I didn't know drinking ever got that serious."

Russell MA, King LE, and Boyd, AS. Lichen Planus after Consumption of a Gold-Containing Liquor. New England Journal of Medicine, 1996; 334:603.

Case shared by:

Lloyd King, M.D.
Professor of Medicine
Vanderbilt University School of Medicine

Michael Zanoli, M.D.
Dermatologist
Heritage Medical Group
Nashville, Tennessee

Chapter Notes

Chapter 1. A *Puzzling Paralysis*
1. Diaz, JH, A 60-year meta-analysis of tick paralysis in the United States; a predictable and often misdiagnosed poisoning. J. Med. Toxicol. 2010. Mar; 6 (1): 15-21.

Chapter 3. The Cause of Some Symptoms Can Be Illusory
Feldman, Marc. *Playing Sick,* Brunner-Rutledge, New York, New York. 2004.
In *Puzzling Symptoms* (C.K. Meador, Cable Publishing, Brule, Wisconsin. 2008), I report additional case reports of several patients with self-harm.

Chapter 12. A Drug to Prevent a Complication Causes the Complication
1. Tomkin GH, Hadden DR, Weaver JA, and Montgomery DAD. Vitamin-B12 Status of Patients on Long-term Merformin Therapy. British Medical Journal, 1971, 2; 685 – 687.

Chapter 14. *An Uncommon Cure*
1. Endocr Pract. 2012 Nov 1;18(6):1038.
Insulinoma in a patient with type 2 diabetes mellitus proved at autopsy.
Kunieda T, Yamakita N, Yasuda K.
2. Dtsch Med Wochenschr. 1988 Nov 4;113(44):1714-7.
[Hypoglycemia caused by insulinoma in diabetes mellitus].

[Article in German]
Heik SC, Klöppel G, Krone W, Iben G, Priebe K, Kühnau J.
3. Diabetes_Complications. 2012 Jan-Feb;26(1):65-7. doi:
10.1016/j.jdiacomp.2011.12.003. Epub 2012 Mar 6.
A rare cause of hypoglycemia in a type 2 diabetic patient: insulinoma.
Cander S, Gül OÖ, Yıldırım N, Unal OK, Saraydaroğlu O, Imamoğlu S.
4. Diabet Med. 2012 Jul;29(7):e133-7. doi: 10.1111/j.1464-
5491.2012.03603.x.
Type 2 diabetes mellitus in a patient with malignant insulinoma manifesting following surgery.
Ademoğlu E, Unlütürk U, Ağbaht K, Karabork A, Corapçioğlu D.

Chapter 16. What You Don't Know Can Kill you.
Howard MA, Hibbard AB, Terrell DR, Medina PJ, Vesely SK, and
George JN; Quinine allergy causing acute severe systemic illness:
report of 4 patients manifesting multiple hematologic, renal, and
hepatic abnormalities. Proc (Baylor University Medical Center).
16 (1): 21-26. 2003.

Chapter 21. Gut Reaction
1. Niederhofer H, Pittschieler K. A preliminary investigation
of ADHD symptoms in persons with celiac disease. *J Atten Disord.*;10(2):200-204. Nov 2006.
2. Addolorato G, Mirijello A, D'Angelo C, et al. Social phobia in
coeliac disease. *Scand J Gastroenterol.* 43(4):410-415. 2008.
3. Ludvigsson JF, Reutfors J, Osby U, Ekbom A, Montgomery SM.
Coeliac disease and risk of mood disorders— a general population-based cohort study. *J Affect Disord.* 99(1-3):117-126. Apr 2007.

Chapter 28. Strange Intuition
1. Johns ME, Moscinski LC, and Sokol L. Phenytoin-associated
Lymphadenopathy Mimicking a Peripheral T-cell Lymphoma.
Mediterr. J. Hematol. Infect. Dis.: 2(2): e20 10028. September 7,
2010. (Published on line).

Biography of
Clifton K.Meador, M.D.

For over fifty years, Clifton K. Meador has been practicing and teaching medicine. This, his thirteenth book, complements his published writings and his well-known satiric articles noting the clinical excesses of modern American medicine, including "The Art and Science of Nondisease," published in the New England Journal of Medicine (1965), "The Last Well Person" also in the New England Journal of Medicine (1994), "A Lament for Invalids" in the Journal of the American Medical Association JAMA 1992) and "Clinical Man: Homo Clinicus," published in Pharos (2011).

His last book True Medical Detective Stories (2012) was dedicated to Berton Roueche, writer for the New Yorker and creator of the genre of medical detective stories.

A graduate of Vanderbilt University in 1955, Dr. Meador has served as executive director of the Meharry Vanderbilt Alliance since 1999, and is an emeritus professor of medicine at both Vanderbilt School of Medicine and Meharry Medical College. Past posts include chief of medicine and chief medical officer of Saint Thomas Hospital (then a major teaching hospital for Vanderbilt) and dean of the University of Alabama School of Medicine.

Dr. Meador lives with his wife, Ann, in Nashville. He is the father of seven, and has seven grandchildren and one great granddaughter.

Made in the USA
Las Vegas, NV
10 April 2023

70429346R00085